T0229332

Conditions Mimicking Asthma

Editor

EUGENE M. CHOO

IMMUNOLOGY AND ALLERGY CLINICS OF NORTH AMERICA

www.immunology.theclinics.com

Consulting Editor
RAFEUL ALAM

February 2013 • Volume 33 • Number 1

ELSEVIER

1600 John F. Kennedy Boulevard • Suite 1800 • Philadelphia, Pennsylvania, 19103-2899

http://www.theclinics.com

IMMUNOLOGY AND ALLERGY CLINICS OF NORTH AMERICA Volume 33, Number 1

February 2013 ISSN 0889–8561, ISBN-13: 978-1-4557-7105-9

Editor: Pamela Hetherington

Immunology and Allergy Clinics of North America (ISSN 0889–8561) is published quarterly by Elsevier Inc., 360 Park Avenue South, New York, NY 10010-1710. Months of issue are February, May, August, and November. Periodicals postage paid at New York, NY and additional mailing offices. Subscription prices are $306.00 per year for US individuals, $442.00 per year for US institutions, $144.00 per year for US students and residents, $375.00 per year for Canadian individuals, $209.00 per year for Canadian students, $547.00 per year for Canadian institutions, $425.00 per year for international individuals, $547.00 per year for international institutions, $209.00 per year for international students. To receive student/resident rate, orders must be accompanied by name of affiliated institution, date of term, and the *signature* of program/residency coordinator on institution letterhead. Orders will be billed at individual rate until proof of status is received. Foreign air speed delivery is included in all *Clinics* subscription prices. All prices are subject to change without notice. **POSTMASTER**: Send address changes to *Immunology and Allergy Clinics of North America*, Elsevier Health Sciences Division, Subscription Customer Service, 3251 Riverport Lane, Maryland Heights, MO 63043. **Customer Service: 1-800-654-2452 (U.S. and Canada); 314-447-8871 (outside U.S. and Canada). Fax: 314-447-8029. E-mail: journalscustomerservice-usa@elsevier.com** (for print support); **journalsonlinesupport-usa@elsevier.com** (for online support).

Reprints. For copies of 100 or more, of articles in this publication, please contact the Commercial Reprints Department, Elsevier Inc., 360 Park Avenue South, New York, New York 10010-1710. Tel. (212) 633-3812, Fax: (212) 462-1935, E-mail: reprints@elsevier.com.

Immunology and Allergy Clinics of North America is covered in MEDLINE/PubMed (Index Medicus), Current Contents/Life Sciences, Science Citation Index, ISI/BIOMED, Chemical Abstracts, and EMBASE/Excerpta Medica.

Printed and bound by CPI Group (UK) Ltd, Croydon, CR0 4YY

Transferred to digital print 2012

Contributors

CONSULTING EDITOR

RAFEUL ALAM, MD, PhD
Professor and Chief, Division of Allergy and Immunology, National Jewish Health, University of Colorado Denver School of Medicine, Denver, Colorado

EDITOR

EUGENE M. CHOO, MD
Assistant Professor of Medicine, Division of Allergy and Immunology, Department of Medicine, National Jewish Health, Denver, Colorado

AUTHORS

KERN BUCKNER, MD
Chief, Division of Cardiology, Professor of Medicine, Department of Medicine, National Jewish Health, Denver, Colorado

EUGENE M. CHOO, MD
Assistant Professor of Medicine, Division of Allergy and Immunology, Department of Medicine, National Jewish Health, Denver, Colorado

FLAVIA C.L. HOYTE, MD
Assistant Professor of Medicine, Division of Allergy and Immunology, Department of Medicine, National Jewish Health, University of Colorado Denver, Denver, Colorado

JOHN R. HURST, PhD, FRCP
Clinical Senior Lecturer, Academic Unit of Respiratory Medicine, Royal Free Campus, UCL Medical School, London, United Kingdom

TODD T. KINGDOM, MD
Department of Otolaryngology, University of Colorado, Aurora, Colorado

ALEX J. MACKAY, MBBS, BSc (Hons), MRCP
Clinical Research Fellow, Academic Unit of Respiratory Medicine, Royal Free Campus, UCL Medical School, London, United Kingdom

ANNYCE MAYER, MD, MSPH
Division of Environmental and Occupational Health Sciences, Department of Medicine, National Jewish Health, Denver; Environmental/Occupational Health, University of Colorado Denver - Colorado School of Public Health, Aurora, Colorado

ALI I. MUSANI, MD, FCCP
Associate Professor of Medicine and Pediatrics, Interventional Pulmonology Program, Division of Pulmonary, Critical Care, Allergy and Immunology; Division of Pulmonary, Critical Care and Sleep Medicine, Department of Medicine, National Jewish Health, Denver, Colorado

KARIN PACHECO, MD, MSPH
Division of Environmental and Occupational Health Sciences, Department of Medicine, National Jewish Health, Denver; Environmental/Occupational Health, University of Colorado Denver - Colorado School of Public Health, Aurora, Colorado

JEEVAN B. RAMAKRISHNAN, MD
Capitol Ear, Nose, and Throat, PA, Raleigh, North Carolina

VIJAY R. RAMAKRISHNAN, MD
Department of Otolaryngology, University of Colorado, Aurora, Colorado

JOSEPH C. SEAMAN, MD
Interventional Pulmonology Program, Division of Pulmonary, Critical Care, Allergy and Immunology, Department of Medicine, National Jewish Health, Denver, Colorado; Lung Associates of Sarasota, Sarasota, Florida

THO TRUONG, MD
Assistant Professor of Medicine, Allergy and Clinical Immunology, National Jewish Health, Denver, Colorado

Contents

Vocal cord dysfunction (VCD), generally characterized by paradoxical closure of the vocal cords during inspiration, is a common mimicker of asthma and of other conditions that cause upper airway obstruction. As a result, it is frequently overlooked and often misdiagnosed, resulting in administration of excessive medications or other unnecessary interventions, with resultant morbidity. This article explores the clinical features, proposed causes, diagnostic considerations, and management of VCD, as well as some differences between VCD and asthma that can aid in differentiating these two diagnoses in the clinical setting.

Tracheobronchomalacia (TBM) and hyperdynamic airway collapse (HDAC) can be debilitating diseases associated with decreased functional capacity and poor quality of life, although there is no standard definition of this complex condition, and there are numerous terms used to describe it. The diverse etiology associated with TBM and HDAC can obscure and delay an accurate diagnosis for years. A thorough medical history is important in understanding possible causes and in guiding diagnostic testing. Medical history may also suggest what treatments may be most beneficial.

Cardiac dyspnea, especially if present only with exercise, is often confused with asthma and exercise-induced bronchospasm. Cardiac dyspnea or asthma is the consequence of pulmonary edema due to pulmonary venous hypertension and not due to asthmatic bronchoconstriction. In overt, acute congestive heart failure, the diagnosis may be readily made by history and physical examination and pertinent laboratory and imaging data.

Anatomy, pathophysiology, epidemiology, and disease characteristics link the upper and lower airways. Nonspecific symptoms such as cough, congestion, shortness of breath, and recurrent infection may be related to the upper airway, lower airway, or both. Patients with the most severe disease often exhibit symptoms and findings of inflammation at both sites. Recent literature suggests that medical treatment and, when appropriate, surgical therapy directed at the upper airway can yield improvements in the lower airway. An understanding of the diagnosis and management of diseases at both sites will afford patients the best possible outcomes.

Bronchiectasis should be considered as a differential diagnosis for, as well as a comorbidity in, patients with asthma, especially severe or long-standing asthma. Chronic airway inflammation is thought to be the primary cause, as with chronic or recurrent pulmonary infection and autoimmune conditions that involve the airways. Consequently, immunodeficiencies with associated increased susceptibility to respiratory tract infections or chronic inflammatory airways also increase the risk of developing bronchiectasis. Chronic bronchiectasis is associated with impaired mucociliary clearance and increased bronchial secretions, leading to airway obstruction and airflow limitation, which can lead to exacerbation of underlying asthma or increased asthma symptoms.

This article describes the different clinical variants of irritant-induced asthma, specifically focusing on high-dose irritant-induced asthma and irritant-induced work-exacerbated asthma, as well as reviews known causes, addresses the often adverse medical and socioeconomic outcomes of this complex condition, and considers issues of causation from an occupational and environmental medicine perspective.

The mechanisms of chronic obstructive pulmonary disease exacerbation are complex. Respiratory viruses (in particular rhinovirus) and bacteria play a major role in the cause of these events. A distinct group of patients seems susceptible to frequent exacerbations, irrespective of disease severity, and this phenotype is stable over time. Many current therapeutic strategies help reduce exacerbation frequency. Further work is required to develop novel anti-inflammatory therapies for exacerbation prevention and treatment. This article focuses on the cause of chronic obstructive pulmonary disease exacerbations, and the current preventative and acute interventions available.

IMMUNOLOGY AND ALLERGY
CLINICS OF NORTH AMERICA

FORTHCOMING ISSUES

May 2013
**Reactions to Aspirin and Other Non-steroidal
Anti-Inflammatory Drugs**
Donald Stevenson and Marek Kowalski,
Editors

August 2013
Exercise-Induced Bronchospasm
Sandra Anderson, *Editor*

November 2013
Angioedema
Bruce Zuraw, *Editor*

ISSUE OF RELATED INTEREST

Clinics in Chest Medicine September 2012 (Volume 33, Number 3)
Asthma
Pascal Chanez, *Editor*

NOW AVAILABLE FOR YOUR iPhone and iPad

Foreword

Conditions Mimicking Asthma

We all see patients who complain of shortness of breath, which is improved with the use of a bronchodilator. The simplest definition of asthma is that it is caused by reversible airway obstruction. Airway obstruction can present with shortness of breath. The improvement with a bronchodilator indicates reversibility. So, is this asthma? Asthma is a syndrome of various pathophysiologic conditions that result in reversible airway obstruction. The latter produces typical symptoms of asthma—shortness of breath, wheezing, and cough. However, none of these symptoms are pathognomic for asthma as they can be elicited by many illnesses of the lungs. As a consequence, many conditions mimic asthma, which leads to misdiagnosis and inappropriate treatment. Bronchial hyperreactivity, as detected by a methacholine test, although a relatively specific and sensitive test, is not foolproof. It is less sensitive in white and nonatopic patients (sensitivity $\sim 77\%$).[1] It is also not very specific when 8 mg/mL concentration of methacholine is used as a cutoff point. At this cutoff level, the positive predictive value of methacholine test is less than 50% (ie, <50% of the subjects in a random population with a PC_{20} <8 mg/mL have clinically current asthma symptoms).[2] Thus, there is no perfect test for asthma. We rely heavily on our clinical judgment. Hence, the consideration of asthma mimickers in our differential diagnoses becomes a top priority. The problem is confounded by the fact that the asthma masqueraders can coexist with asthma in the same patient. Thus, the proper diagnosis of asthma and its masqueraders, and determination of their relative contribution to the clinical presentation, if they co-exist, is extremely important.

Asthma management can be further complicated by comorbidities that aggravate asthma or one of its symptoms. The diagnosis of asthma confounders and their proper treatment play an essential role in optimal management of asthma. To address this important topic of asthma masqueraders and confounders, I have asked my colleague Dr Eugene Choo to lead the way. He has invited an excellent group of experts and put together a comprehensive list of articles that will surely enrich our knowledge and improve our practice.

Rafeul Alam, MD, PhD
Division of Allergy and Immunology
National Jewish Health and
University of Colorado Denver School of Medicine
1400 Jackson Street
Denver, CO 80206, USA

E-mail address:
alamr@njc.org

Supported by NIH grants RO1 AI091614 and AI68088, PPG HL36577, and N01 HHSN272200700048C.

Immunol Allergy Clin N Am 33 (2013) ix–x
http://dx.doi.org/10.1016/j.iac.2012.11.005
0889-8561/13/$ – see front matter © 2013 Published by Elsevier Inc.
immunology.theclinics.com

REFERENCES

1. Sumino K, Sugar EA, Irvin CG, et al, American Lung Association Asthma Clinical Research Centers. Methacholine challenge test: diagnostic characteristics in asthmatic patients receiving controller medications. J Allergy Clin Immunol 2012;130: 69–75.e6.
2. Cockcroft DW. Direct challenge tests: Airway hyperresponsiveness in asthma: its measurement and clinical significance. Chest 2010;138(Suppl 2):18S–24S.

Preface

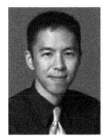

Eugene M. Choo, MD
Editor

Asthma is one of the most common diseases seen by physicians in the field of allergy and immunology. Although this diagnosis is often solely made on a clinical basis, particularly by primary care physicians, objective confirmation is frequently obtained by evaluating for bronchodilator reversibility or bronchial hyperreactivity. In most cases, an initial clinical suspicion for asthma is correct.

However, invariably we will come across patients that were initially given a diagnosis of asthma, but whose presentations now suggest that another process may be responsible for some, if not all, of their signs and symptoms. Suspicion for another disease may be raised by a number of factors: an unusual constellation of symptoms, a characteristic symptom trigger, disease severity out of proportion to pulmonary function testing, or failure to respond to usual treatment regimens. The importance of correctly identifying the presence of another etiology is critical, as a misdiagnosis can result in years of poorly controlled symptoms and reduced quality of life, not to mention a chronic asthma medication regimen that is then unnecessary or ineffective.

Although many conditions could potentially mimic or contribute to asthma, the emphasis here is on the most common etiologies likely to be encountered by clinicians. This issue of *Immunology and Allergy Clinics of North America* contains contributions from various experts on these mimickers of asthma, spanning the specialties of allergy/immunology, pulmonology, otolaryngology, occupational/environmental medicine, and cardiology. Discussion of other eosinophilic lung diseases, such as allergic bronchopulmonary aspergillosis/mycosis or Churg-Strauss syndrome, will be the specific focus of a future issue.

In this issue, Flavia Hoyte discusses vocal cord dysfunction, including its clinical features, proposed causes, diagnostic considerations, and management. As a frequent cause of incorrectly diagnosed "refractory" asthma, it is an important factor to consider.

Tho Truong highlights bronchiectasis and immunodeficiency, two conditions that can occur independently or concurrently in patients with or without asthma.

Jeevan Ramakrishnan, Todd Kingdom, and Vijay Ramakrishnan bring their otolaryngology expertise to bear on the issue of allergic rhinitis and chronic rhinosinusitis.

Immunol Allergy Clin N Am 33 (2013) xi–xii
http://dx.doi.org/10.1016/j.iac.2012.12.001
0889-8561/13/$ – see front matter © 2013 Published by Elsevier Inc.
immunology.theclinics.com

The contribution of these diseases to lower respiratory symptoms and the unified airway theory are emphasized.

Kern Buckner focuses on cardiac causes of dyspnea, particularly on aspects of cardiac disease that would be most relevant to allergy/immunology physicians in clinical practice.

Annyce Mayer and Karin Pacheco offer suggestions on reactive airways dysfunction syndrome, discussing how irritants and work-related exposures can impact respiratory symptoms and asthma.

In conjunction with Joseph Seaman and Ali Musani, I summarize tracheobronchomalacia and hyperdynamic airway collapse: its pathophysiology, clinical presentation, diagnostic evaluation, and treatment options. This diagnosis is important and often delayed for years; it is likely to become more frequent as contributing factors such as obesity increase in prevalence.

Finally, chronic obstructive pulmonary disease (COPD) is discussed in an article that was initially presented in a previous issue. COPD is always an important consideration given its large amount of potential overlap with asthma.

I hope that this issue will stimulate awareness and potentially improve diagnosis and management of these important conditions.

Eugene M. Choo, MD
Division of Allergy and Immunology
National Jewish Health
1400 Jackson Street
Denver, CO 80206, USA

E-mail address:
chooe@njhealth.org

Vocal Cord Dysfunction

Flavia C.L. Hoyte, MD

KEYWORDS

- Vocal Cord Dysfunction (VCD) • Paradoxical Vocal Cord Motion (PVCM)
- Asthma Mimicker • Vocal Cord

KEY POINTS

- Vocal cord dysfunction (VCD) is a disorder that goes by many names and can vary in presentation from patient to patient.
- VCD is a common mimicker of asthma, and both conditions frequently coexist.
- The current mainstay of VCD treatment is speech therapy and the elimination of possible triggers for upper airway hyperreactivity, most notably upper airway inflammation and gastroesophageal reflux disease.
- Although these interventions are effective in many patients with VCD, there are refractory cases for whom a paucity of reasonable therapeutic options exist.

INTRODUCTION

Vocal cord dysfunction (VCD), a term that refers to inappropriate adduction of the vocal cords during inhalation and sometimes exhalation, is a functional disorder of the vocal cords that serves as an important mimicker of asthma.[1–4] As discussed later, there are many terms that have been used interchangeably with VCD, sometimes with minor differences between terms. To avoid confusion, the term VCD is used in this article to refer to the group of conditions that encompasses all of these terms. Patients with VCD are often misdiagnosed as having asthma, allergies, or severe upper airway obstruction. Many of these patients have been treated with excessive medications or other unnecessary interventions, with resultant morbidity, as a result of misdiagnosis. The misclassification of patients with VCD is likely a result of the many gaps that still remain in our understanding of VCD, as well as the similarities between the clinical presentation of VCD and these other conditions. This article explores the clinical features, proposed causes, diagnostic considerations, and management of VCD as well as some differences between VCD and asthma that can aid in differentiating these 2 diagnoses in the clinical setting.

HISTORICAL PERSPECTIVE

Although VCD has received increasing attention over the past several decades, the first reports of this condition came under various different names in the nineteenth

Division of Allergy and Immunology, Department of Medicine, National Jewish Health, 1400 Jackson Street, Denver, CO 80206, USA
E-mail address: hoytef@njhealth.org

Immunol Allergy Clin N Am 33 (2013) 1–22
http://dx.doi.org/10.1016/j.iac.2012.10.010
0889-8561/13/$ – see front matter © 2013 Elsevier Inc. All rights reserved.
immunology.theclinics.com

century.[5] In 1842, Dunglison described "hysteric croup" as dysfunction of the laryngeal muscles sometimes seen in hysterical women.[6] In that same year, Austin Flint included a description of 2 men with a similar presentation in his textbook *Principles and Practice of Medicine* and termed their condition "laryngismus stridulus."[7] The first case of VCD noted on laryngoscopy was in 1869 by MacKenzie, who again made the diagnosis in "hysteric" patients.[8] In 1902, Sir William Osler described VCD as a disorder that could affect both the inspiratory and expiratory phases of the respiratory cycle in the textbook *The Principles and Practice of Medicine*.[9] It was not until 70 years later that VCD made its next appearance in the medical literature, this time termed "Munchausen's stridor" in a case report by Patterson and colleagues[10] regarding a 33-year-old woman with recurrent episodes of acute dyspnea and stridor that had led to 15 hospital admissions and were attributed to dysfunction of the vocal cords. Since then, there have been more than 70 terms used to describe VCD or similar conditions.[11]

TERMINOLOGY

As alluded to earlier, VCD was initially believed to be seen only in the context of psychological illness or hysteria. In addition to the 3 terms already mentioned, VCD believed to be primarily caused by a psychological component has been referred to as emotional laryngeal wheezing,[12] psychogenic upper airway obstruction,[13] and psychogenic stridor.[14] Over the past several decades, the recognition that VCD can occur outside psychological illness has shifted the medical literature toward more general terms such as pseudoasthma,[15] nonorganic upper airway obstruction,[16] functional upper airway obstruction,[17] factitious asthma,[18] spasmodic croup,[19] episodic laryngeal dyskinesia,[20] functional laryngeal obstruction,[21] functional laryngeal stridor,[22] episodic paroxysmal laryngospasm,[23] irritable larynx syndrome (ILS),[24] and paradoxic vocal fold motion (PVFM).[25] Of these terms, the most common are VCD, which is most often used by pulmonologists, allergists, and mental health practitioners, and PVFM, more popular among otolaryngologists and speech-language pathologists.[5] A recent *Clinics* article by Christopher and Morris delineates the terms VCD, PVFM, and intermittent arytenoid region prolapse (IARP), also known as functional laryngomalacia. The investigators propose that these 3 conditions can be lumped together under an umbrella term POLO, which stands for periodic occurrence of laryngeal obstruction, a term that emphasizes that all 3 conditions lead to functional, rather than organic, obstruction of the upper airway and therefore present similarly. The main difference between these 3 entities is that VCD and PVFM occur at the level of the glottis, whereas IARP occurs at the supraglottic level and is less associated with cough.[5] As noted by Christopher and Morris in their *Clinics* article, PVFM would be a misnomer in cases of expiratory VCD, in which inappropriate adduction of the vocal cord structures during exhalation leads to upper airway obstructive symptoms, because the inappropriate vocal fold motion is not technically paradoxic because vocal cord adduction can occur during normal exhalation. These investigators choose the term VCD rather than PVFM, as the more inclusive term of the 2, and we do the same here for the sake of simplicity.[5] However, when approaching patients with symptoms of VCD, it is important to keep in mind the plausibility of VCD subgroups and the broad differential diagnosis of VCD, in particular organic or anatomic causes of upper airway obstruction that are not strictly functional in nature.

CLINICAL PRESENTATION

VCD is a transient obstruction of the upper airway associated with the paradoxic adduction or closure of the vocal folds (or cords). Although it occurs primarily during inhalation, VCD can occur during either or both stages of the respiratory cycle.[4,26–29] The clinical presentation of VCD ranges from no symptoms to mild dyspnea to acute respiratory distress, which can be mistaken for an asthma attack.[30] Patients typically complain of acute-onset breathing difficulty, tightness localized to the throat, and in some cases stridor or laryngeal wheezing.[29,31,32] Dyspneic events may be described as air hunger or a sensation of choking and can be frightening, eliciting panic and anxiety in some patients, a response that tends to perpetuate the dysfunctional vocal cord movement and worsen the respiratory symptoms. Additional symptoms, which are variable among patients, can include chest tightness or pain, difficulty swallowing, a globus pharyngeus sensation, intermittent aphonia or dysphonia, neck or chest retractions, fatigue, or throat clearing during episodes. Most patients have a concomitant chronic cough.[29,31,33] One theory, proposed by Vernigan and colleagues,[34] speculates that chronic cough and VCD are linked and are different manifestations of a single underlying condition. They constructed a model depicting chronic cough and VCD on a continuum, with pure cough at one end, pure VCD on the other, and some combination of the 2 in the middle.

VCD episodes frequently begin and end abruptly,[35] and specific triggers can only sometimes be identified. Self-reported triggers may include one or several of the following: upper respiratory infections, occupational exposures, talking, laughing, singing, acid reflux, cough, foods, physical exertion, exercise, postnasal drip, weather changes, emotional stressors, odors, strong scents, and other airborne irritants.[24,31] Some patients show a priming effect, whereby they move from having a single trigger to gradually being triggered by multiple, previously benign, agents. If VCD is triggered in a large group setting, it can set off a mass hysterialike reaction, sometimes as a result of an identifiable noxious exposure[36,37] and sometimes as a result of a contagious hysteria with no obvious trigger.[5,38]

EPIDEMIOLOGY

Once believed to be a psychiatric disorder of women between 20 and 40 years of age, particularly those with a medical background and victims of previous abuse,[1] VCD is now believed to affect a broader patient base. A literature review by Brugman and colleagues[39] of 1530 patients with VCD found that 65% of these patients were adults, classified as older than 19 years of age, but that the remainder were children and adolescents. The age range of these patients was broad, ranging from 0.02 to 82 years, with a median age of 36.5 years for the adults in the group and 14 years for the pediatric patients. For all age groups, there was a 3:1 female predominance. Although this female predominance was also found in another literature review of 1161 patients with VCD by Morris and colleagues,[40] the female/male ratio in this study was found to be only 2:1. The initially proposed increased incidence of VCD in patients with a medical background or an underlying psychological dysfunction has also been brought into question by Brugman's extensive review of the literature.[39]

Although some investigators have attempted to capture the prevalence of VCD through literature review and retrospective study,[39–41] its true incidence remains unknown. In a prospective study of 1025 patients with dyspnea as their chief complaint, Kenn and colleagues[42] found VCD in 2.8% of their sample. Another study by Ciccolalla and colleagues[43] looked retrospectively at 236 patients admitted to an inner city hospital asthma center for an asthma exacerbation and found 4 VCD diagnoses, resulting in an incidence of roughly 2%. In 1994, Newman and Dubester[4] studied a subset of asthmatics with refractory asthma and found a higher incidence of VCD, with nearly 10% of their patients having VCD alone and an additional 30%

of their patients having both VCD and asthma. Like adults, children with severe asthma were also found to have a high rate of VCD in a study by Gavin and colleagues,[44] which determined the incidence to be around 14%. The rates of VCD reported for nonasthmatic teens and young adults are more variable, ranging from 8%[45] in 1 study to 15%[46] and 27%[47] in 2 other studies. Overall, VCD is a diagnosis that is likely underappreciated in clinical practice, and a large prospective study of the general population would be necessary to establish its true incidence.

LARYNGEAL PHYSIOLOGY

The 3 basic functions of the larynx are protection, respiration, and phonation, all of which are regulated at least in part by involuntary brainstem reflexes. Of these functions, only the protective function is strictly reflexive and involuntary, whereas the other 2 functions can be initiated voluntarily.[48]

The most important function of the larynx is pulmonary protection, which is mediated primarily by the glottic closure reflex and the cough reflex. Together, these reflexes protect the airway from potentially noxious inhaled stimuli and prevent aspiration of foreign material during respiration and of food and liquid particles during eating and drinking.[48–50] In addition to cough and glottic closure, other reflex responses to irritant stimuli include mucous secretion, sneeze, apnea, and increased bronchomotor tone.[51]

Glottic closure is mediated by the superior laryngeal nerve, the recurrent laryngeal nerve, and the vagal nerve.[51] These nerves mediate closure of the 3 layers of the laryngeal structure. The first layer involves coordination of the aryepiglottic folds, the epiglottis, and the arytenoid cartilages. To form this layer, the aryepiglottic folds come together to cover the superior inlet of the larynx, the epiglottis inverts to protect the anterior gap, and the arytenoid cartilages protect the posterior gap. The second layer of laryngeal protection is mediated by closure of the true vocal folds, and the third layer is provided by forceful adduction of the false vocal folds.[48]

The cough reflex is generally initiated by an adverse stimulus triggering one of several sensory receptors, resulting in afferent information being sent to the brainstem.[50] Laryngeal sensory receptors were categorized by Brugman into 4 functional categories: (1) cold receptors that respond to changes in temperature; (2) irritant receptors that respond to mechanical deformation, as well as to irritants and aerosols; (3) pressure receptors that respond to changes in laryngeal transmural pressure; and (4) drive receptors that respond to laryngeal motion. The irritant receptors are considered the main players in the glottis closure and cough reflexes.[11] The sensory receptors of the airway are believed to be distributed in a specific manner, with more mechanosensitive receptors proximally and more chemosensitive receptors distally.[50]

The vocal cords abduct, or open, widely during quiet breathing in both normal individuals and those with asthma. Glottic widening during inhalation is consistent between individuals and begins just before the onset of inspiratory flow, reaching a maximum width at midinspiration. Inspiratory laryngeal movements are shown in **Fig. 1** for patients with and without VCD.

Unlike inspiratory movement, movement of the vocal cords during exhalation can vary significantly between individuals. In a normal individual, the vocal cords generally adduct, or close, between 10% and 40% of their aperture, beginning at end inspiration and continuing until approximately two-thirds of vital capacity has been expelled.[4]

CAUSE

The cause of VCD is believed to vary from one patient to the next, dependent in large part on which comorbidities are present. Several considerations should be

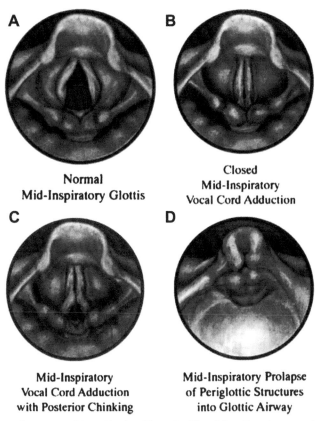

A Normal Mid-Inspiratory Glottis

B Closed Mid-Inspiratory Vocal Cord Adduction

C Mid-Inspiratory Vocal Cord Adduction with Posterior Chinking

D Mid-Inspiratory Prolapse of Periglottic Structures into Glottic Airway

Fig. 1. Vocal cord movement in patients with and without functional upper airway obstruction. (*A*) Normal vocal cord appearance at midinspiration. (*B*) Paradoxic adduction of the vocal cords during midinspiration, as seen in most cases of VCD. (*C*) Partial adduction of the vocal cords with posterior chinking, as seen in a small percentage of VCD cases. (*D*) Prolapse of the periglottic structures, as seen in IARP, also known as functional laryngomalacia. (*Data from* Hicks M, Burgman S, Katial R. Vocal cord dysfunction/paradoxic vocal fold motion. Prim Care Clin Office Pract 2008;35:85.)

taken into account as potential contributing factors that lead to paradoxic movement of the vocal folds. These factors include psychological, physiologic, and neurologic considerations.

Psychological Considerations

Since the 1800s when VCD was first described as hysteric croup by Dunglison, this disorder has been closely tied to psychological factors.[52] This association was perpetuated by several case studies from the 1970s and early 1980s, as well as a case series published by Christopher and colleagues[1] in 1983. In this study, the investigators found that 4 of the 5 patients with documented VCD had psychiatric comorbidities, ranging from "mild stress-related exacerbation of symptoms to obsessive-compulsive disorder." These investigators noted varying degrees of secondary gain in all of the patients and suggested that they might be suffering from a conversion disorder.[1] Similarly, in a review by Lacy and McManis in the late 1990s,[53] 45 of 48 patients with VCD carried one of several psychiatric diagnoses, the most common of which were a conversion disorder (52%), major depression (13%), factitious disorder (10%), obsessive-compulsive disorder (4%), and adjustment disorder (4%). Although both of these studies suggest that VCD may be the result of a conversion disorder, this has never been definitively proved and is no longer the current thinking. Other stressors such as physical abuse, sexual abuse, depression, family stress, and posttraumatic stress resulting from a combat environment have all been linked to VCD.[32]

Although Brugman[39] found psychological factors present in 39% of the 1530 patients that she reviewed in 2003, she did not find data to support a preponderance of abuse. Others have described similar findings of patients with VCD who lack an emotional or psychiatric disturbance,[26,32,54] and some investigators suggest that the depression and anxiety often seen in these patients is a result of their chronic respiratory illness, rather than a cause.[4,26,32]

Physiologic Considerations

The most likely cause of VCD is laryngeal hyperresponsiveness, which can be caused by a variety of irritant and nonirritant triggers. The sensory receptors described earlier, which mediate the cough and glottic closure reflexes, are found in the larynx, trachea, and larger airways.[50] Stimulation of these sensory receptors can occur directly or indirectly, via olfactory nerve stimulation or direct stimulation of sensory nerve endings in the upper and lower respiratory tract. These nerves trigger local reflex arcs or more complex nerve signals involving the brain and brainstem, leading to closure of the vocal folds when exposed to such triggers.[51] It has been suggested that the glottic closure reflex may be accentuated in patients with VCD, causing various extrinsic and intrinsic stimuli to trigger reflex closure of the vocal cords in a manner generally reserved for protection of the airway against harmful exposures.[50] In 1999, Morrison and colleagues[24] defined the ILS, which is essentially upper airway hyperresponsiveness that results from chronic noxious stimulation. Such chronic stimulation, they theorized, results in changes to the laryngeal control region of the brainstem, leading to hyperexcitability of the neuronal networks controlling the larynx, which yields hyperresponsiveness of vocal cords and resultant VCD.

Aside from ambient irritant triggers, which are variable from patient to patient, gastroesophageal reflux disease (GERD) and postnasal drip tend to be the most common causes of laryngeal inflammation and hyperresponsiveness. Gastric reflux and upper airway secretions have both been implicated in the apnea of infants as a result of hyperresponsive laryngeal chemoreflexes.[55,56] Canine models of GERD have indicated that a pH of 2.5 or less provokes laryngospasm through vagally mediated mechanisms and the sensitization of mucosal chemoreceptors.[57]

In their continuum between VCD and cough, Vernigan and colleagues[34] proposed that gastroesophageal reflux and postnasal drip are among the underlying causes linking these 2 conditions. In their study of 78 patients with chronic cough, Palombini and colleagues[58] proposed a pathogenic triad of asthma, postnasal drip syndrome, and GERD as the most frequent causative factors of chronic cough. Their findings were in accordance with 4 other published studies that revealed the same results in most chronic cough cases. A subsequent review of the literature by Altman and colleagues[50] found that 86% of adult patients with chronic cough had allergic rhinitis, cough-variant asthma, or GERD as the cause of their cough. These investigators found that patients with upper airway hypersensitivity are more prone to develop cough in response to a variety of irritant stimuli targeting the upper and lower airways. Viral upper respiratory infections, irritant inhalation (eg, noxious gases and fumes, smoke), gastroesophageal reflux, laryngopharyngeal reflux (LPR), postnasal drip, and exercise have all been associated with cough and VCD.[26,39,46,59–61]

A large study by Bucca and colleagues[62] of 441 nonasthmatic patients with symptoms of wheeze, sudden attacks of dyspnea, and nonproductive cough revealed that 67% of these patients had upper airway hyperresponsiveness, as defined by a 25% decrease in maximal midinspiratory flow during histamine inhalation challenge. Concurrent upper respiratory tract diseases were assessed, and the following were found to be common: postnasal drip (55%), pharyngitis (55%), laryngitis (40%), and sinusitis (32%).[62] The correlation between these inflammatory conditions, upper airway hyperresponsiveness as shown by testing, and the symptoms of VCD suggests that inflammation of the upper airway and larynx is likely a key player in the development of upper airway hyperresponsiveness, leading to an enhanced glottis closure reflex and to paradoxic adduction of the vocal cords on inspiration, as seen in VCD.

Neurologic Considerations

Maschka and colleagues[63] have described several organic causes of VCD, which include disorders that cause brainstem compression (Arnold-Chiari malformation and cerebral aqueductal stenosis), severe cortical or upper motor neuron injury (cerebral vascular accidents and static encephalopathy), nuclear or lower motor neuron injury (amyotrophic lateral sclerosis, myasthenia gravis, and medullary infarction), and movement disorders (adductor laryngeal breathing dystonia (ALBD), myoclonic disorders, parkinsonism syndromes, and drug-induced brainstem dysfunction). In addition to these many secondary neurologic causes of VCD, Harbison and colleagues[54] described 2 cases of stridor caused by PVFM after thyroidectomy. Both cases were believed to be caused by laryngeal trauma during surgery and endotracheal intubation, as well as a temporary palsy of the recurrent laryngeal nerve as a result of surgical manipulation. Ayres and Gabbott proposed that alterations in the autonomic nervous system might contribute to upper airway hyperresponsiveness and subsequent VCD.[64] In their theory, an inflammatory product, such as a virus or allergic rhinitis, would trigger an afferent signal from the larynx to a more central brain region, which includes sites in the medulla, midbrain, and the prefrontal cortex. Areas 25 and 32 of the brain, in particular, are polysynaptically linked with the larynx and have a strong potential to influence autonomic function. Through such a pathway, the initial inflammatory insult might lead to an autonomic preset that would allow subsequent stimuli (such as psychological stressors or changes in ambient temperature) to induce parasympathetic reflexes, leading to airway narrowing in either the upper or lower airways. This situation would result in an exaggeration of the protective role of the larynx and to VCD after previously benign exposures.[64]

DIFFERENTIAL DIAGNOSIS

The most common symptoms of VCD are episodic dyspnea, cough, and wheezing,[29,40] symptoms that can accompany diseases of either the upper or lower airways.[11] The broad differential diagnosis listed in **Table 1** is important when evaluating a patient with possible VCD because VCD can coexist with many of these other conditions, sometimes confounding diagnosis.

APPROACH TO THE PATIENT WITH POSSIBLE VCD

A detailed assessment of patients with suspected VCD generally involves each of the following: clinical history and physical examination, pulmonary testing, measures of oxygenation, and flexible laryngoscopy. The importance placed on each individual

Table 1 Differential diagnosis of VCD	
Diagnostic Categories	Examples
Infectious	Epiglottitis, bronchiolitis, laryngotracheobronchitis (croup), laryngitis, pharyngeal abscess, diphtheria, pertussis, laryngeal papillomatosis
Rheumatologic	Rheumatoid cricoarytenoid arthritis, relapsing polychondritis, laryngeal sarcoidosis
Neoplastic	Cancer of the head and neck, cystic hygroma, hemangioma, rhabdomyosarcoma, teratoma, lymphoma, papilloma
Endocrine	Thyroid goiter
Traumatic	Laryngeal injury or fracture, thermal injury, upper airway hemorrhage, caustic ingestion
Allergic	Angioedema, anaphylaxis, exercise-induced anaphylaxis
Neurologic	Brainstem anomalies, vocal cord paralysis or paresis, tic disorders, multiple sclerosis, postpolio syndrome, multiple system atrophy, myasthenia gravis, Meige syndrome, Gerhardt disease, Parkinson disease, diaphragmatic flutter syndrome, respiratory spasmodic dysphonia, traction on the recurrent laryngeal nerve, true laryngospasm
Pulmonary	Asthma, exercise-induced bronchoconstriction, chronic obstructive pulmonary disease, foreign body aspiration, hyperventilation syndrome, pulmonary embolus
Congenital	Laryngomalacia, laryngeal cleft, intrathoracic vascular ring, subglottic stenosis, laryngeal web
Psychiatric	Conversion disorder, Münchausen syndrome, malingering, panic disorders, anxiety disorder, somatization disorder
Gastrointestinal	GERD, LPR
Occupational	Gulf War laryngotracheitis, World Trade Center cough, inhalational injury
Other	Goiter, benign cysts, spasmodic croup

Adapted from Hicks M, Burgman S, Katial R. Vocal cord dysfunction/paradoxic vocal fold motion. Prim Care Clin Office Pract 2008;35:86.

area varies depending on whether the patient is presenting with chronic symptoms or experiencing an acute exacerbation. The comprehensive approach to patients with possible VCD is summarized in **Box 1**, and each of the 4 components of assessment is discussed later in greater detail.

Clinical History and Physical Examination

A careful clinical history may provide valuable information in diagnosing VCD.[11,65] A targeted line of questioning around pertinent features of VCD, such as specific signs, symptoms, and predisposing factors, may help distinguish VCD from other respiratory conditions, including asthma.[11] These features are summarized in **Box 2** and include several of the symptoms and predisposing factors discussed in the earlier sections on clinical presentation and cause.

Many of the signs and symptoms listed in **Box 2** can help direct suspicion toward the upper airway as the area of the dysfunction, and patients often point to or grab their throat when describing their respiratory symptoms.[50,65] Hyperventilation is common among patients with VCD, leading to symptoms of lightheadedness, visual

Box 1
Approach to the patient with possible VCD

1. Clinical History and Physical Examination

   a. Questions regarding symptoms

      i. Do you have more trouble getting air in or getting air out?
      ii. Do you feel any tightness?
      iii. If so, where is the tightness located (throat, upper chest, lower chest)?
      iv. Do you hear any noises when you breathe in?
      v. When symptoms start, do you generally cough?
      vi. Do you ever lose your voice or have a change in the way your voice sounds?
      vii. Do you have numbness or tingling in your hands, feet, or lips during episodes?
      viii. Do you ever feel lightheaded or dizzy?
      ix. Have you ever passed out or felt as though you were going to pass out?
      x. Do symptoms come on rapidly?
      xi. Do symptoms resolve rapidly?
      xii. Do asthma medications help?
      xiii. Does use of your asthma inhalers sometimes make symptoms worse?

   b. Assessing for potential risk factors or laryngopharyngeal irritants

      i. GERD/LPR
      ii. Postnasal drip because of upper airway inflammatory conditions
      iii. Psychological factors
      iv. Other risk factors listed in **Box 2**

   c. Physical examination

      i. Rule out upper airway obstruction from an organic cause
      ii. Look for signs of upper airway inflammation or allergic rhinitis
      iii. Look for signs of acute VCD: stridor, tachypnea, hoarseness, or dysphonia, cough, tugging of the neck or upper chest muscles, and a look of anxiety or even distress

   d. Response to treatment

      i. During acute episode, no improvement or even worsening with inhaled medications
      ii. During chronic management, lack of response to escalating asthma therapy including corticosteroids

2. Pulmonary Function Testing

   a. Inspiratory flow loop that is often poorly reproducible and truncated, saw-toothed, or irregular
   b. FEF_{50} (forced expiratory flow at 50% of the exhaled vital capacity)/FIF_{50} (forced inspiratory flow at 50% of the inhaled vital capacity) greater than 1
   c. If FEV_1 (FEV in first second of expiration) is reduced, FEV_1/FVC (forced vital capacity) ratio is normal
   d. Normal lung volumes

3. Measure of Oxygenation and Ventilation During Episodes

   a. Pulse oximetry normal
   b. Normal oxygen tension measured on arterial blood gas (Pao_2 [partial pressure of oxygen, arterial])
   c. Normal alveolar-arterial (A-a) gradient
   d. Reduced arterial Pco_2 (partial pressure of carbon dioxide) because of hyperventilation

4. Flexible Laryngoscopy

   a. Paradoxic adduction of vocal cords during inhalation
   b. Posterior chinking
   c. Inappropriate adduction of vocal cords during exhalation
   d. Secondary evidence of postnasal drip/GERD/LPR (edema and erythema of the glottic or periglottic region)

Box 2
Important aspects of the clinical history in a patient with VCD

1. Symptoms of VCD
   a. Throat or upper chest tightness
   b. Shortness of breath or dyspnea
   c. Sensation of choking or suffocation
   d. More difficulty getting air in than out
   e. Cough
   f. Lightheadedness or dizziness
   g. Heavy sensation of the extremities
   h. Perioral or extremity numbness or tingling
   i. Rapid onset and rapid resolution of these symptoms
2. Signs of VCD
   a. Tachypnea or hyperventilation
   b. Stridor
   c. Neck or chest retractions
   d. Pallor but no cyanosis
   e. Hoarseness or dysphonia
   f. Lack of relief, and sometimes worsening, from asthma inhalers
3. Risk Factors for VCD
   a. Upper airway inflammation (allergic or nonallergic rhinitis, chronic sinusitis, recurrent upper respiratory infections)
   b. GERD
   c. Previous traumatic event involving breathing (eg, suffocation, near-drowning, witnessing a severe asthma attack)
   d. Severe emotional distress
   e. Female gender
   f. Playing a wind instrument
   g. Competitive athletics

---

changes, numbness, or tingling in 76% of patients with VCD in a study by Parker and colleagues.[66] Hyperventilation likely accounts for related symptoms of extremity heaviness, dizziness, and near-syncope or syncope sometimes described by these patients. Patients with VCD who have been treated for asthma often report that metered dose or powder inhalers can trigger or exacerbate their symptoms, whereas nebulized medications provide relief.[50] This situation may be a result of the method of delivery for these medications. Inhalers require patients to hold their breath before exhaling, which could exacerbate VCD, whereas nebulized treatments are administered as the patient breathes calmly, deeply, and evenly for 5 to 15 minutes.[67]

Examination of the oropharynx and upper airway is essential to eliminate other causes of upper airway obstruction, including organic causes, which can indicate a more serious underlying condition and sometimes require immediate treatment.[11,40,52] Actively looking for signs of upper airway inflammation, such as cobblestoning of the oropharynx, postnasal drip, swollen turbinates, nasal polyps, allergic shiners, or pharyngeal erythema, can help identify underlying processes such as rhinitis, sinusitis, and even GERD or LPR that might be contributing to laryngeal hypersensitivity and resultant VCD in a given patient.[11] From a respiratory standpoint, the examination of patients with VCD is generally unrevealing unless they are actively symptomatic. However, during attacks, VCD often presents with stridor, tachypnea, hoarseness or dysphonia, cough, tugging of the neck or upper chest muscles, and a look of anxiety or even distress.[68]

Pulmonary Testing

A characteristic finding of nonorganic extrathoracic airway obstruction is a highly variable, nonreproducible, and abnormal configuration of the inspiratory loop during spirometry, as shown in **Fig. 2**.[11,51]

Flattening or truncation of the inspiratory flow loop and irregularities such as a sawtoothed pattern can be observed during an acute VCD attack,[4,50,51] but also when patients are asymptomatic.[29] Because similar abnormalities can also be seen in other laryngeal disorders, clinical context becomes crucial in differentiating disorders of the larynx.[50] Importantly, organic causes of upper airway obstruction often serve as a fixed obstruction and yield blunting of both the inspiratory and expiratory loops, which should prompt a radiologic and endoscopic evaluation looking for a fixed obstructive process rather than for a functional disorder like VCD.[4] In contrast to inspiratory VCD, asthma and expiratory VCD generally causes truncation or scooping of the expiratory loop on spirometry.[51,69,70]

One useful spirometric measure for assessing patients with VCD is the FEF_{50}/FIF_{50} ratio, which is normally less than or equal to 1. However, in patients with predominantly inspiratory VCD, this ratio is usually greater than 1 because of truncation of the inspiratory loop, which reduces the FIF_{50}.[11,50,71] A ratio of greater than 1 is not always

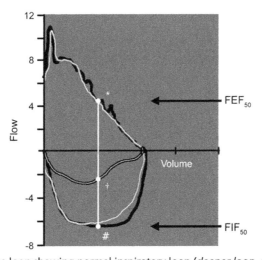

Fig. 2. Flow-volume loop showing normal inspiratory loop (*deeper loop, marked with hash*) and the truncated inspiratory loop of VCD (*flattened loop, marked with dagger*). The FEF_{50} is marked with an asterisk. The FIF_{50} is marked with a hash on the normal inspiratory loop and with dagger on the VCD inspiratory loop. The FEF_{50}/FIF_{50} ratio is normally less than 1, as shown by the ratio of asterisk to hash. In VCD, the FEF_{50}/FIF_{50} ratio is usually greater than 1, as shown by the ratio of asterisk to dagger. (*Data from* Hicks M, Burgman S, Katial R. Vocal cord dysfunction/paradoxic vocal fold motion. Prim Care Clin Office Pract 2008;35:90.)

observed when inspiratory VCD is accompanied by expiratory obstruction,[11,40,50] and this ratio may be difficult to interpret in cases of VCD with comorbid asthma.[11]

When performing full pulmonary function tests with lung volumes in a patient with VCD but no asthma, one should see normal lung volumes because they do not experience air trapping. Accordingly, patients with pure VCD have normal chest radiographs with no indication of hyperinflation.[50] This finding is in contrast to patients with asthma who generally show signs of air trapping, such as hyperinflation on chest radiographs and enlarged lung volumes, in particular the residual volume, during pulmonary function testing.

Methacholine and histamine, commonly used to trigger airway hyperreactivity as part of an evaluation for asthma, have also been used as irritant stimuli to invoke a VCD attack.[26,72] Bucca and colleagues[73] showed that a greater than 25% decrease in the maximum inspiratory flow during histamine inhalation challenge was associated with changes in midinspiratory glottic area. Patients with VCD frequently show evidence of inappropriate vocal fold movement during the inspiratory or expiratory phase of breathing when a laryngoscopy is performed immediately after a methacholine challenge. This finding is in contrast to patients who do not have VCD or to those patients who have VCD but are asymptomatic during laryngoscopy and often show normal vocal cord movement.[51] Bronchial provocation with methacholine has a high negative predictive value and can therefore be helpful in ruling out a diagnosis of asthma.[74] If successful in triggering a VCD attack during methacholine challenge, performing a laryngoscopy immediately after a bronchial challenge can help determine whether a patient has asthma, VCD, neither diagnosis, or both.

Some patients' VCD attacks are not triggered by methacholine, so a negative laryngoscopy in an asymptomatic patient does not rule out the diagnosis of VCD, as alluded to earlier. If methacholine challenge fails to elicit VCD in patients with a compelling history, a specific challenge to a known irritant, ideally performed in a challenge chamber under close observation, may be indicated.[51,75] Provocation with exercise is required to elicit symptoms in those patients with exercise-induced VCD.[4,27,46]

Measures of Oxygenation and Ventilation During Episodes

Even during an acute attack, patients with VCD do not show cyanosis and are able to maintain normal oxygenation, as measured by pulse oximetry or arterial blood gas sampling, distinguishing VCD from several other causes of respiratory distress.[1,11] The alveolar-arterial oxygen difference (P_{AO_2}-P_{aO_2}), also known as the A-a gradient, is a measure of oxygen delivery, and is normal at less than 10 mm Hg in patients with VCD, even during attacks.[1] This finding is in contrast to acute asthma attacks, which causes the A-a gradient (P_{AO_2}-P_{aO_2}) to increase as a result of P_{aO_2} reduction, which occurs in direct proportion to the degree of airflow limitation as an asthma attack progresses.[69] During a VCD attack, on the other hand, the P_{aO_2} is generally normal, with one notable exception: breath holding. If breath holding occurs during a VCD attack, the P_{aO_2} is reduced, but one also sees an increased P_{aCO_2}, which is unusual in VCD. In general, the P_{aCO_2} of patients with VCD is low rather than high, because of the hyperventilation that accompanies most VCD attacks. In a study by Parker and colleagues,[66] an end-tidal CO_2 of less than 30 mm Hg, a physiologic consequence of hyperventilation, was seen in 48% of the patients with VCD studied.

Flexible Laryngoscopy

Direct visualization of the vocal folds via flexible, transnasal fiber-optic laryngoscopy during an acute attack remains the gold standard for diagnosis of VCD.[11,26,29,40,41] Unlike the respiratory symptoms caused by an acute asthma attack, VCD attacks do not usually impede panting, speaking, or taking deep breaths.[11] Hence, patients should be instructed to perform various maneuvers during laryngoscopy, including sequential phonation, normal breathing, panting, and repetitive deep breaths, to assess vocal cord movement in a comprehensive manner.[4,40]

Newman and colleagues[29] reported findings diagnostic of VCD in 100% of patients undergoing laryngoscopy while symptomatic and in 60% of patients who were asymptomatic at the time of evaluation. Christopher and colleagues[1] were the first to depict the classically described laryngoscopic findings shown in **Fig. 1**, including paradoxic adduction of the membranous portion of the vocal folds and the presence of a diamond-shaped posterior glottic chink during the inspiratory, expiratory, or both cycles of breathing. In a review of the literature, Brugman found complete inspiratory vocal fold adduction at midinspiration to be the most common laryngoscopic finding, present in 66% of adult and pediatric patients with VCD, and glottic chinking to be present in only 5% of these patients.[39] Inspiratory closure of the vocal folds is considered sufficient for diagnosis. Caution is advised to avoid anesthetizing the vocal folds or stimulating the posterior pharynx during examination, because this could yield false results.[40]

VCD occurring exclusively during expiration is uncommon[11,40] and should be diagnosed with caution. Expiratory glottic closure can be observed in normal individuals and exaggerated in asthmatics during exercise or during bronchospasm, as might be seen after a bronchial challenge. The laryngeal positive end expiratory pressure (auto PEEP), is a compensatory mechanism seen in acute asthma attacks as a way of prolonging expiration, thereby increasing intrathoracic pressures and maintaining higher lung volumes to prevent alveolar collapse.[41,51,65] The glottic narrowing during expiration that allows for auto PEEP can be misinterpreted as expiratory VCD in patients with bronchial hyperreactivity that has been triggered by the prelaryngoscopy bronchial challenge.

VCD AS A MIMICKER OF ASTHMA

Patients with VCD are typically misdiagnosed as having refractory asthma, with resultant mistreatment.[29] A review of the literature by Morris and colleagues[40] found that 32.7% of the 1161 patients with VCD whom they reviewed were misdiagnosed with asthma before the appropriate diagnosis of VCD was made. When administered pharmacologic treatment of asthma, patients with VCD generally do not improve and frequently have side effects or iatrogenic complications of high-dose corticosteroids, bronchodilators, intubation, and tracheostomy.[29,41,46,76] In a study of 95 adult patients with VCD, Newman and colleagues[29] found that patients were misdiagnosed with asthma for an average of 4.8 years before being diagnosed with VCD. During this time, they were treated with medications identical to patients with severe asthma, including daily prednisone in 81% of these patients, with an average dose of 29.2 mg daily. These patients averaged 9.7 emergency room visits and 5.9 admissions in the year before presentation, and 28% of the patients had been intubated. Similarly, in a retrospective study by Andrianopoulos and colleagues[31] of 27 patients referred for VCD and related syndromes, 90% had been placed on numerous pharmacologic agents to treat their symptoms, with the most frequent incorrectly prescribed medications being bronchodilators in 52% of patients and systemic steroids in 44%. Approximately 25% of patients in this second study received emergency room treatment and inpatient hospitalization, whereas only 7% of them had undergone intubation or tracheostomy.

In addition to minimizing unnecessary tests, treatments, and morbidity associated with an incorrect diagnosis, identifying cases of VCD early can help decrease the psychological effects of this diagnosis and improve the long-term prognosis for patients.[76] Given the serious consequences of misdiagnosis, it is therefore important to differentiate VCD from asthma. One complicating factor in doing so is the fact that VCD can coexist with adult and pediatric asthma and with exercise-induced broncho-constriction.[11,29,46,66] The rate of VCD as a comorbidity of asthma has been estimated at 38% in adult asthmatics and 40% in pediatric patients with asthma.[29,65] **Table 2** shows several clinical features that can help distinguish VCD from asthma.

TREATMENT OF VCD

Management of VCD is guided by the comorbidities that are present in a given patient and requires a multidisciplinary approach. The team may include the primary care physician, pulmonologist, allergist, otolaryngologist, gastroenterologist, neurologist, psychiatrist/psychologist, speech-language pathologist, athletic coach, or athletic trainer.[50,59,77]

Patient education is an important component of treatment, beginning with careful and compassionate disclosure of the diagnosis. The patient should be educated on normal laryngeal anatomy and physiology as it relates to breathing, vocalizing, swal-lowing, coughing, throat clearing, and breath holding. They should then be taught about the paradoxic or otherwise inappropriate movement of the vocal folds under stress or when exposed to specific triggers, as well as during an acute VCD attack. If the VCD was diagnosed by laryngoscopy, viewing the videotape or DVD further enhances understanding and acceptance and can even allow the patient to visualize overcoming the laryngeal obstruction with breathing exercises, if such maneuvers were captured as part of the endoscopic evaluation.[11] Knowledge of both normal physiology and the functional abnormalities that are causing their symptoms can help empower patients to accept and gain control over this disorder.

For patients previously misdiagnosed with asthma, unnecessary medications should be discontinued gradually and under the care of physician, especially in patients in whom underlying airway hyperreactivity has not been ruled out.[1,32,40] In those individuals with coexisting asthma who may have been overtreated as a result of previously undiagnosed VCD, medications can generally be tapered.[69] Pharmaco-logic treatment and lifestyle modifications should be used if the medical team is able to

Table 2 Differentiating VCD from asthma		
	Asthma	VCD
Gender (female/male ratio)	1:1	3:1
Location of tightness	Chest	Neck/throat
Stridor vs wheeze	Wheeze	Stridor
Inspiratory vs expiratory symptoms	Expiratory	Inspiratory
Response to asthma therapy	Yes	No
Nocturnal symptoms	Yes	No
Refractory period	Yes	No
Late-phase response	Yes	No
Symptom onset during exercise	>10 min	<5 min
Recovery period after exercise	15–60 min	5–10 min

Adapted from Hicks M, Burgman S, Katial R. Vocal cord dysfunction/paradoxic vocal fold motion. Prim Care Clin Office Pract 2008;35:87.

identify specific airway irritants, such as gastroesophageal reflux, LPR, allergic and nonallergic rhinitis, chronic sinusitis, or recurrent upper respiratory infections.[32]

Acute Management

The acute management of VCD requires a confirmed diagnosis, and treatment should be directed toward relieving the airway obstruction.[40] The first step is to reassure the patient that the condition is benign and that their oxygen levels are normal despite the intense dyspnea, and to calmly validate their fears.[2,11,40] Morris and colleagues[40] found that reassurance alone is effective at relieving the acute airway symptoms of VCD. Various maneuvers such as panting, nasal inhalation or sniffing, and pursed-lip breathing on exhalation, can serve to open the upper airway and possibly abort VCD attacks.[21,31,70,78]

Medications can also play a role in the treatment of acute VCD attacks. Heliox, a mixture of helium and oxygen, is available in helium/oxygen ratios of 80:20, 70:30, and 60:40[79] and has been found to be dramatically effective in relieving acute presentations of VCD,[1,71,79–82] but not in all cases.[38,83] Helium, which has a lower density than nitrogen, allows the oxygen in heliox to flow through occluded large airways more easily than ambient air would, by producing less turbulent flow.[40,80] Enhancing oxygen delivery in this manner reduces the work of breathing and ideally helps patients feel more at ease so that they eventually allow their vocal folds to relax.[80] In severe cases, sedation can be used in the acute setting, because symptoms nearly always disappear with sleep or anxiolysis.[11] Accordingly, benzodiazepines have proved effective in terminating acute VCD episodes.[40] A more invasive and rarely used treatment approach involves intralaryngeal injection of botulinum toxin type A. This toxin acts by preventing acetylcholine release at nerve endings, resulting in chemical denervation, which paralyzes the vocal fold in the open position.[11,30,40] Although this technique has been used to successfully treat ALBD and spasmodic dystonia,[11,32] a review by Morris and colleagues in 2006[40] found only 9 reported cases of botulinum toxin used to treat VCD. Given the obvious risks associated with paralyzing the vocal cords in an open position, this therapy should be considered only for individuals with severe protracted VCD who are unresponsive to all other therapies and are seriously considering intubation or tracheostomy.[11,30,52]

Chronic Management

Speech therapy, which consists of a detailed assessment followed by comprehensive treatment, is regarded as the primary treatment of VCD.[4,11,29,35,41,53,69,71] Speech therapists, also known as vocal pathologists, play an important role in long-term management of VCD by providing assessment and diagnostic input as well as the following therapeutic interventions: patient education, supportive counseling, management/suppression of laryngeal abusive behaviors (ie, cough and throat clearing), voice therapy, respiratory retraining, and desensitization to specific irritants.[32,35,51] In addition to speech therapy, patients may also benefit from psychological counseling.[40] Although psychotherapy lacks systematic study as a therapeutic intervention in VCD,[11,32,40] it may be warranted in patients whose VCD is believed to be worsened by stress or related to an underlying psychiatric condition.[32,84] Electroencephalographic neurofeedback, basic biofeedback, surface electromyography biofeedback, and hypnosis have been reported as effective in some adolescents with VCD.[27,84–89]

Speech-Language Pathology Assessment

Assessment by a speech-language pathologist generally begins with a comprehensive patient interview to understand the patient's knowledge of their symptoms and reason for referral. Discrepant, inconsistent, or underappreciated information can emerge from this assessment.[32] Before initiating speech therapy, for example, many patients are unaware that speech-language pathologists also specialize in diseases and disorders of the larynx, including upper airway obstruction and respiration. In addition, for many patients with newly diagnosed VCD, the diagnosis is one that they have never heard of previously. Often, VCD replaces a different diagnosis, such as asthma, that a patient has carried for many years. Most patients have received medications for their previous diagnosis and are now being told to wean or even discontinue these medications. Together, these factors can generate skepticism about the diagnosis of VCD. In this respect, it is important to find out a given patient's background and history.

In addition to establishing a patient's background, the initial case history should explore the specifics of a given patient's VCD to target therapy to that particular patient. Helpful historical clues include specific symptoms; triggers; associated psychosocial features such as anxiety or panic; methods currently being used by the patient to resolve their symptoms; effect of inhalers (when prescribed); changes in vocal quality; changes in swallowing; existence of laryngeal abusive behaviors such as throat clearing or coughing; presence of laryngopharyngeal irritants (eg, postnasal drip, GERD, or LPR); and lifestyle factors that might be contributing to the disorder (eg, hydration practices, breathing patterns, and vocal habits). Referrals to other physicians or counselors are sometimes made as indicated by this comprehensive interview.

Speech-Language Pathology Treatment

The type of therapy provided by the speech-language pathologists at National Jewish Health is outlined later. However, treatment of VCD must be tailored to the specific needs of a given patient and any one treatment may not be helpful or sufficient in all cases.

As described earlier, an important part of speech therapy is education. Patients are instructed about the pathophysiology of VCD, including hypersensitivity of the larynx and hyperactivity of the normal protective function of the vocal folds. They are then educated on the role of laryngeal abusive behaviors (eg, cough and throat clearing) in VCD and are provided with techniques to eliminate these behaviors, as well as the rationale behind doing so.

Patients are taught various breathing techniques, collectively known as quick-release techniques because they serve to rapidly release the vocal folds from the paradoxic movement that is responsible for the symptoms of VCD. These techniques, which are summarized in **Box 3**, were developed by a revered voice pathologist from National Jewish Health, Fran Lowry.[68]

Speech therapy techniques are ideally tailored to meet the needs of each patient on an individualized basis. Patients who have a tendency toward hyperventilation or who have significant anxiety or panic, for example, are instructed on controlled breathing exercises. These exercises focus on a more controlled pursed-lip breathing pattern using abdominal support, with focus directed at relaxation. Once the optimal technique is determined for a given patient, they are encouraged to practice 5 repetitions of the technique, 20 times a day, when asymptomatic and to use the technique at the first onset of difficulty. Practicing the technique repeatedly not only assists with laryngeal relaxation and retraining but also ensures that patients can eventually respond automatically with these techniques during times of need.[68]

Quick-release techniques can be used either for prevention of VCD attacks or for control of such attacks. To maximize the benefit of these techniques, patients are encouraged to recognize triggers for their episodes, so that they might use a given

---

Box 3
Speech therapy techniques used for relief of VCD symptoms

1. Relaxed throat breathing with abdominal support
   a. Lower shoulders
   b. Place hand on midabdomen to support it
   c. Breathe gently in through nose and make sure abdomen comes out
   d. Breathe gently out through slightly pursed lip and make sure abdomen comes in
   e. Ensure that breathing is comfortable and easy so that there is no tugging of the torso or neck muscles

2. Quick Inhalation
   a. Inhale quickly through the nose or mouth for approximately 1 second
   b. Use caution with rapid inhalation through the nose in patients with sinus disease or postnasal drip, so as not to trigger cough or throat clearing because of secretions
   c. Causes forced abduction of the vocal cords

3. Pursed-Lip Breathing
   a. Breathe out slowly through pursed lips (as if to whistle) for 2 to 3 seconds
   b. Ensure that what is being inhaled is also being exhaled
   c. Focus on timing to make sure that exhalation is not too long, which generates tension rather than relieving it
   d. Pursed-lip breathing slows down the breathing rate and creates pressure behind the lips and throughout the pharynx to forcibly abduct the vocal cords

---

technique as soon as they realize that they have been exposed to a known trigger instead of waiting for the onset of symptoms. If a patient does not recognize that they have been exposed or cannot identify specific triggers, they should at least use quick-release techniques at the time of their first symptom to abort the attack as early as possible. By providing immediate release of the vocal folds, these techniques can decrease the anxiety and panic that often accompany VCD attacks. After learning these techniques, many patients are successful in preventing or controlling attacks, sometimes as early as their first speech therapy session.[68]

Quick-release techniques are also used for desensitization to specific irritants and to prevent or control VCD attacks brought on by exercise. With the help of a specific irritant challenge, patients whose VCD attacks are brought on by irritant exposures can undergo progressive desensitization such that they can control and frequently prevent episodes. Exercise challenges can be used in a similar fashion for patients with exercise-induced VCD. The type of exercise used in the challenge should mimic as closely as possible the exercise known to set off a patient's symptoms, and the setting of the challenge should resemble the environment in which this exercise generally takes place (eg, indoors vs outdoors). For those athletes who push their bodies to physiologic limits and beyond, therapy is directed at relieving upper and lower body tension and reversing maladaptive patterns such as shallow breathing, poor posture, and breath holding. Paced breathing techniques, with a focus on using abdominal support and recognizing the initial onset of symptoms, can be useful in exercise-induced VCD. At the first onset of symptoms, patients are taught to use the quick-release techniques and to maintain their pace steadily. If symptoms do not resolve at this pace, they decrease their pace until symptoms resolve. Once symptoms subside, patients gradually increase their pace and continue to focus on their breathing.[68]

SUMMARY

VCD is a disorder that goes by many names and can vary in presentation from patient to patient. Although VCD was first recognized in the mid-1800s, it remains underappreciated and misdiagnosed in clinical practice. VCD is a common mimicker of asthma, and both conditions frequently coexist. It is imperative that the medical community gains a better understanding of VCD and increases awareness of the condition to avoid unnecessary morbidity from misdiagnosis and the inappropriate therapeutic interventions that often follow. The current mainstay of VCD treatment is speech therapy and the elimination of possible triggers for upper airway hyperreactivity, most notably upper airway inflammation and GERD. Although these interventions are effective in many patients with VCD, there are refractory patients for whom a paucity of reasonable therapeutic options exist.

ACKNOWLEDGMENTS

Thank you to Rohit Katial, MD for his assistance in the preparation of this article. Thank you also to Janson Ainsworth for his administrative support.

REFERENCES

1. Christopher KL, Wood RP, Eckert C, et al. Vocal cord dysfunction presenting as asthma. N Engl J Med 1983;308:1566–70.
2. Bahrainwala AH, Simon MR. Wheezing and vocal cord dysfunction mimicking asthma. Curr Opin Pulm Med 2001;7:8–13.
3. Mobeireek A, Alhamad A, Al-Subaei A, et al. Psychogenic vocal cord dysfunction simulating bronchial asthma. Eur Respir J 1995;8:1978–81.
4. Newman KB, Dubester SN. Vocal cord dysfunction: masquerader of asthma. Semin Respir Crit Care Med 1994;15(2):161–7.
5. Christopher KL, Morris MJ. Vocal cord dysfunction, paradoxic vocal fold motion, or laryngomalacia? Our understanding requires an interdisciplinary approach [review]. Otolaryngol Clin North Am 2010;43(1):43–66, viii.
6. Dunglison RD. The practice of medicine. Philadelphia: Lea and Blanchard; 1842. p. 257–8.
7. Flint A. Principles and practice of medicine. Philadelphia: Lea and Blanchard; 1842. p. 267–8.
8. MacKenzie M. Use of laryngoscopy in diseases of the throat. Philadelphia: Lindsey and Blackeston; 1869. p. 246–50.
9. Osler W. Hysteria. In: Osler W, editor. The principles and practice of medicine. 4th edition. New York: Appleton; 1902. p. 1111–22.
10. Patterson R, Schatz M, Horton M. Munchausen's stridor: non-organic laryngeal obstruction. Clin Allergy 1974;4:307–10.
11. Brugman SM. What's this thing called vocal cord dysfunction. Available at: http://www.chestnet.org/education/online/pccu/vol20/lessons25. Accessed July 30, 2007.
12. Rodenstein DO, Francis C, Stanescu DC. Emotional laryngeal wheezing: a new syndrome. Am Rev Respir Dis 1983;127:354–6.
13. Barnes SD, Grob CS, Lachman BS, et al. Psychogenic upper airway obstruction presenting as refractory wheezing. J Pediatr 1986;109(6):1067–70.

14. Lund DS, Garmel GM, Kaplan GS, et al. Hysterical stridor: a diagnosis of exclusion. Am J Emerg Med 1993;11(4):400–2.
15. Dailey RH. Pseudoasthma: a new clinical entity? JACEP 1976;5(3):192–3.
16. Cormier YF, Camus P, Desmeules MJ. Non-organic acute upper airway obstruction: description and a diagnostic approach. Am Rev Respir Dis 1980;121(1): 147–50.
17. Appelblatt NH, Baker SR. Functional upper airway obstruction. A new syndrome. Arch Otolaryngol 1981;107(5):305–6.
18. Downing ET, Braman SS, Fox MJ, et al. Factitious asthma: physiological approach to diagnosis. JAMA 1982;248:2878–81.
19. Collett PW, Brancatisano T, Engel LA. Spasmodic croup in the adult. Am Rev Respir Dis 1983;127(4):500–4.
20. Ramírez J, León I, Rivera LM. Episodic laryngeal dyskinesia. Clinical and psychiatric characterization. Chest 1986;90(5):716–21.
21. Pitchenik AE. Functional laryngeal obstruction relieved by panting. Chest 1991; 100(5):1465–7.
22. Smith ME, Darby KP, Kirchner K, et al. Simultaneous functional laryngeal stridor and functional aphonia in an adolescent. Am J Otol 1993;14(5):366–9.
23. Gallivan GJ, Hoffman L, Gallivan KH. Episodic paroxysmal laryngospasm: voice and pulmonary function assessment and management. J Voice 1996;10(1): 93–105.
24. Morrison M, Rammage L, Emami AJ. The irritable larynx syndrome. J Voice 1999; 13(3):447–55.
25. Patel NJ, Jorgensen C, Kuhn J, et al. Concurrent laryngeal abnormalities in patients with paradoxical vocal fold dysfunction. Otolaryngol Head Neck Surg 2004;130(6):686–9.
26. Perkner JJ, Fennelly KP, Balkissoon R, et al. Irritant-associated vocal cord dysfunction. J Occup Environ Med 1998;40(2):136–43.
27. McFadden ER, Zawadski DK. Vocal cord dysfunction masquerading as exercise-induced asthma: a physiologic cause for "choking" during athletic activities. Am J Respir Crit Care Med 1996;153:942–7.
28. Reisner C, Nelson HS. Vocal cord dysfunction with nocturnal awakening. J Allergy Clin Immunol 1997;99:843–6.
29. Newman KB, Mason UG III, Schmaling KB. Clinical features of vocal cord dysfunction. Am J Respir Crit Care Med 1995;152:1382–6.
30. Maillard I, Schweizer V, Broccard A, et al. Use of botulinum toxin type A to avoid tracheal intubation or tracheostomy in severe paradoxical vocal cord movement. Chest 2000;118:874–7.
31. Andrianopoulos MV, Gallivan GJ. PVCM, PVCD, EPL, and irritable larynx syndrome: what are we talking about and how do we treat it. J Voice 2000; 14(4):607–18.
32. Mathers-Schmidt BA. Paradoxical vocal fold motion: a tutorial on a complex disorder and the speech-language pathologist's role. Am J Speech Lang Pathol 2001;10:111–25.
33. Diamond E, Kane C, Dugan G. Presentation and evaluation of vocal cord dysfunction. Chest 2000;118(4):199S.
34. Vernigan AE, Theodoros DG, Gibson PG, et al. The relationship between chronic cough and paradoxical vocal fold movement: a review of the literature. J Voice 2006;20(3):466–80.
35. Vlahakis NE, Patel AM, Maragos NE, et al. Diagnosis of vocal cord dysfunction: the utility of spirometry and plethysmography. Chest 2002;122:2246–9.

36. Jones TF, Craig AS, Hoy D, et al. Mass psychogenic illness attributed to toxic exposure at a high school. N Engl J Med 2000;342:96–100.
37. Cairns-Pastor C. Condition has name, but still unsettling. Tampa Tribune; 2003.
38. Arndt GA, Voth BR. Paradoxical vocal cord motion in the recovery room: a masquerader of pulmonary dysfunction. Can J Anaesth 1996;43(12): 1249–51.
39. Brugman S. The many faces of vocal cord dysfunction: what 36 years of literature tell us. Am J Respir Crit Care Med 2003;167:A588.
40. Morris MJ, Allan PF, Perkins PJ. Vocal cord dysfunction: etiologies and treatment. Clin Pulm Med 2006;13:73–86.
41. Patterson DL, O'Connell EJ. Vocal cord dysfunction: what have we learned in 150 years. Insights in Allergy 1994;9(6):1–9.
42. Kenn K, Willer G, Bizer C, et al. Prevalence of vocal cord dysfunction in patients with dyspnea: first prospective clinical study. Am J Respir Crit Care Med 1997; 155:A965.
43. Ciccolella DE, Brennan KJ, Borbely B, et al. Identification of vocal cord dysfunction (VCD) and other diagnoses in patients admitted to an inner city university hospital asthma center. Am J Respir Crit Care Med 1997;155:A82.
44. Gavin LA, Wamboldt M, Brugman S, et al. Psychological and family characteristics of adolescents with vocal cord dysfunction. J Asthma 1998;35(5):409–17.
45. Abu-Hasan M, Tannous B, Weinberger M. Exercise-induced dyspnea in children and adolescents: if not asthma then what? Ann Allergy Asthma Immunol 2005;94: 366–71.
46. Morris MJ, Deal LE, Bean DR, et al. Vocal cord dysfunction in patients with exertional dyspnea. Chest 1999;116(6):1676–82.
47. Seear MD, Wensley DW, West N. How accurate is the diagnosis of exercise-induced asthma amongst Vancouver schoolchildren? Arch Dis Child 2005; 90(9):898–902.
48. Sasaki CT, Weaver EM. Physiology of the larynx. Am J Med 1997;103:9S–18S.
49. O'Hollaren MT. Dyspnea originating from the larynx. Immunol Allergy Clin North Am 1996;16(1):69–76.
50. Altman KW, Simpson CB, Amin MR, et al. Cough and paradoxical vocal fold motion. Otolaryngol Head Neck Surg 2002;127(6):501–11.
51. Balkissoon R. Occupational upper airway disease. Clin Chest Med 2002;23: 717–25.
52. Weiss TM. Vocal cord dysfunction: paradoxical vocal cord motion–a thorough review. Available at: http://www.utmb.edu/otoref/grnds/Vocal-Cord-2001-07/VCD-2htm. Accessed January 17, 2007.
53. Lacy TJ, McManis SE. Psychogenic stridor. Gen Hosp Psychiatry 1994;16: 213–23.
54. Harbison J, Dodd J, McNicholas WT. Paradoxical vocal cord motion causing stridor after thyroidectomy. Thorax 2000;55:533–4.
55. Thach BT. Reflux associated apnea in infants: evidence for a laryngeal chemoreflex. Am J Med 1997;103:120S–4S.
56. Orenstein SR. An overview of reflux-associated disorders in infants: apnea, laryngospasm, and aspiration. Am J Med 2001;111:60S–3S.
57. Loughlin CJ, Koufman JA, Averill DB. Acid-induced laryngospasm in a canine model. Laryngoscope 1996;106(12):1506–9.
58. Palombini BC, Castilhos Villanova CA, Araujo E, et al. A pathogenic triad in chronic cough: asthma, postnasal drip syndrome, and gastroesophageal reflux disease. Chest 1999;116:279–84.

59. Murry T, Tabaee A, Aviv JE. Respiratory retraining of refractory cough and laryngopharyngeal reflux in patients with paradoxical vocal fold movement disorder. Laryngoscope 2004;114:1341–5.
60. Taramarcaz P, Grissell TV, Borgas T, et al. Transient postviral vocal cord dysfunction. J Allergy Clin Immunol 2004;114(6):1471–2.
61. Suttithawil W, Chakkaphak S, Jaruchinda P, et al. Vocal cord dysfunction concurrent with a nutcracker esophagus and the role of gastroesophageal reflux disease. Ann Allergy Asthma Immunol 2006;96:373–5.
62. Bucca C, Rolla G, Brussino L, et al. Are asthma-like symptoms due to bronchial or extrathoracic airway dysfunction. Lancet 1995;346:791–5.
63. Maschka DA, Bauman NM, McCray PB, et al. A classification scheme for paradoxical vocal fold motion. Laryngoscope 1997;107(11):1429–35.
64. Ayres JG, Gabbot PLA. Vocal cord dysfunction and laryngeal hyperresponsiveness: a function of altered autonomic balance. Thorax 2002;57:284–5.
65. Martin RJ, Blager FL, Gay ML, et al. Paradoxic vocal cord motion in presumed asthmatics. Semin Respir Med 1987;8(4):332–7.
66. Parker JM, Berg BW. Prevalence of hyperventilation in patients with vocal cord dysfunction. Chest 2002;122S:185S–6S.
67. Medline plus. Drug information: albuterol inhalation. Available at: http://www.nlm.nih.gov/medlineplus/druginfo/meds/a682145.html. Accessed on October 28th, 2012.
68. Hicks M, Brugman SM, Katial R. Vocal cord dysfunction/paradoxical vocal fold motion [review]. Prim Care 2008;35(1):81–103.
69. Brugman SM, Newman K. Vocal cord dysfunction. Medical/Scientific Update 1993;11(5):1–6.
70. Bahrainwala AH, Simon MR, Harrison DD, et al. Atypical expiratory flow volume curve in an asthmatic patient with vocal cord dysfunction. Ann Allergy Asthma Immunol 2001;86:439–43.
71. Goldman J, Muers M. Vocal cord dysfunction and wheezing. Thorax 1991;46:401–4.
72. Perkins PJ, Morris MJ. Vocal cord dysfunction induced by methacholine challenge testing. Chest 2002;122:1988–93.
73. Bucca C, Rolla G, Scappaticci E, et al. Histamine hyperresponsiveness of the extrathoracic airway in patients with asthmatic symptoms. Allergy 1991;46:147–53.
74. Crapo RO, Casaburi R, Coates AL, et al. Guidelines for methacholine and exercise challenge testing–1999. This official statement of the American Thoracic Society was adopted by the ATS Board of Directors, July 1999. Am J Respir Crit Care Med 2000;161(1):309–29.
75. Stanton AE, Bucknall CE. Vocal cord dysfunction. Breathe 2005;2(1):31–7.
76. Hayes JP, Nolan MT, Brennan N, et al. Three cases of paradoxical vocal cord adduction followed up over a 10-year period. Chest 1993;104(3):678–80.
77. Sandage MJ, Zelazny SK. Paradoxical vocal fold motion in children and adolescents. Lang Speech Hear Serv Sch 2004;35:353–62.
78. Blager FB. Paradoxical vocal fold movement: diagnosis and management. Curr Opin Otolaryngol Head Neck Surg 2000;8:180–3.
79. Weir M. Vocal cord dysfunction mimics asthma and may respond to heliox. Clin Pediatr 2002;41(1):37–41.
80. Borish L. Acute workup of vocal cord dysfunction. Ann Allergy Asthma Immunol 2003;91:318.
81. Gose JE. Acute workup of vocal cord dysfunction. Ann Allergy Asthma Immunol 2003;91:318.

82. Weir M, Ehl L. Vocal cord dysfunction mimicking exercise-induced broncho-spasm in adolescents. Pediatrics 1997;99:923–4.
83. Wood RP, Blager FB, Milgrom H. Vocal cord dysfunction mimicking exercise-induced bronchospasm in adolescents. Pediatrics 1997;99:923–4.
84. Anbar RD, Hehir DA. Hypnosis as a diagnostic modality for vocal cord dysfunc-tion. Pediatrics 2000;106(6):1–3.
85. Warnes E, Allen KD. Biofeedback treatment of paradoxical vocal fold motion and respiratory distress in an adolescent girl. J Appl Behav Anal 2005;38:529–32.
86. Ferris RL, Eisele DW, Tunkel DE. Functional laryngeal dyskinesia in children and adults. Laryngoscope 1998;108:1520–3.
87. Nahmias J, Tansey M, Karetzky MS. Asthmatic extrathoracic upper airway obstruction: laryngeal dyskinesia. Niger J Med 1994;91:616–20.
88. Smith MS. Acute psychogenic stridor in an adolescent athlete treated with hypnosis. Pediatrics 1983;72:247–8.
89. Caraon P, O'Toole C. Vocal cord dysfunction presenting as asthma. Ir Med J 1991;84:98–9.

Tracheomalacia/ Tracheobronchomalacia and Hyperdynamic Airway Collapse

Eugene M. Choo, MD[a],*, Joseph C. Seaman, MD[b],
Ali I. Musani, MD, FCCP[c]

KEYWORDS

- Tracheomalacia • Tracheobronchomalacia • Hyperdynamic airway collapse
- Excessive dynamic airway collapse • Airway stenting • Trachoebronchoplasty

KEY POINTS

- Tracheomalacia/tracheobronchomalacia (TBM) and hyperdynamic airway collapse (HDAC) are distinct diseases with significant clinical overlap.
- TBM involves loss of structural integrity of cartilaginous structures of the airway wall, whereas HDAC is an exaggeration of normal airway-wall movement with luminal intrusion of the posterior membrane.
- Both TBM and HDAC can mimic asthma and should be suspected in individuals with symptoms disproportional to an initial diagnosis, or in patients who fail to respond to appropriate treatment for this diagnosis.
- Diagnostic evaluation includes chest computed tomography with dynamic expiratory imaging, pulmonary function tests, and the gold standard of bronchoscopy. Treatment includes aggressive medical management of contributing causes (whether inflammatory or mechanical) and comorbid conditions.
- If symptoms persist, trial of airway stenting is indicated to identify individuals who should receive definitive surgical correction with tracheobronchoplasty.

INTRODUCTION

Tracheomalacia/tracheobronchomalacia (TBM) and hyperdynamic airway collapse (HDAC) can cause respiratory signs and symptoms that result in significant functional impairment and reduced quality of life. TBM and HDAC result in loss of structural

Disclaimers: None.
[a] Division of Allergy and Immunology, Department of Medicine, National Jewish Health, 1400 Jackson Street, Denver, CO 80206, USA; [b] Interventional Pulmonary, Pulmonary, and Critical Care Lung Associates of Sarasota, 1921 Waldemere Street, Suite 705, Sarasota, FL 34239, USA; [c] Interventional Pulmonology Program, Division of Pulmonary, Critical Care, Allergy and Immunology, Department of Medicine, National Jewish Health, 1400 Jackson Street, Denver, CO 80206, USA
* Corresponding author.
E-mail address: ChooE@NJHealth.org

integrity of the airway walls and have similar clinical presentations but distinct areas of affected anatomy. Because of their clinical presentation and diversity of potential causes, it is fairly easy for symptoms to be mistakenly attributed to asthma or other disorders, delaying accurate diagnosis for years.[1]

DEFINITION

Although they are often not clearly distinguished, TBM and HDAC have different definitions (albeit with significant overlap).[2] In addition, they frequently coexist in the same patient. Strictly speaking, tracheomalacia signifies diffuse or segmental weakness of the trachea. Tracheobronchomalacia refers to tracheomalacia that has extension into one or both mainstem bronchi. The terms tracheomalacia and TBM are often used indiscriminately, and therefore in this article are simply termed TBM unless necessary.[3] In TBM there is loss of structural integrity of the cartilaginous structures of the airway wall. When changes in airway pressure occur (such as with forced expiratory maneuvers or coughing), these hypermobile cartilaginous structures, which are normally curved, flatten.[1,2]

HDAC, also known as excessive dynamic airway collapse, consists of exaggeration of normal airway-wall movement, and involves airway compromise caused by intrusion of the posterior membrane. Normal individuals with structurally uncompromised airways can have up to 35% narrowing of the airway lumen with forced expiratory maneuvers or coughing,[2,4] and this is deemed abnormal when collapse of the airways with forced expiratory maneuvers is greater than 50%.[1,2] TBM and HDAC may coexist in some severe cases, with patients having incompetence of cartilaginous structures as well as posterior membrane invagination.[1,2]

EPIDEMIOLOGY

The prevalence of TBM and HDAC is unclear; studies have yet to be performed in general populations. In select study populations, prevalence has been highly variable owing to differences in diagnostic definitions and testing modalities.

The incidence of TBM and HDAC was found to range from 4% to 23% in patients with various respiratory symptoms undergoing video-bronchoscopy.[1,2,5,6] In one study looking at 163 patients receiving evaluation for possible pulmonary embolism, 16 (10%) met the criteria for TBM.[7] TBM and HDAC seem to be most common in men older than 40 years, at least in early reports.[6]

NATURAL HISTORY

TBM and HDAC are typically progressive diseases. Jokenan and colleagues[6] found worsening of airway narrowing in 76% of a case series of 17 TBM patients on repeat bronchoscopy. In a larger study looking at patients with tracheomalacia, TBM, or bronchomalacia, Nuutinen[8] followed 94 patients for 5.2 years. Most patients who received repeat bronchoscopy showed worse disease, and none improved. Among patients with progression, 6 of 9 tracheomalacia patients worsened to TBM, and all 5 subjects with bronchomalacia deteriorated to TBM.[3]

HISTOPATHOLOGY

There is a dearth of detailed information regarding histopathology in TBM and HDAC, but in general it depends on the underlying etiology. TBM involves incompetence of cartilaginous airway structures, and this is also where the main abnormalities are found. In one case series, the ratio of cartilage rings to soft tissue was reduced or even absent altogether, impairing the structural integrity of the airway.[2]

On the other hand, as HDAC involves posterior membrane invagination into the airway lumen, this posterior portion of the airway membrane is either unable to maintain normal tone or is simply redundant.[2] In normal airways, this posterior portion moves posteriorly during inhalation, which increases the size of the airway lumen. To prevent excessive distention, longitudinal smooth muscle fibers tighten. The posterior membranous portion moves forward into the airway lumen during exhalation, with longitudinal smooth-muscle fibers tightening to prevent excessive airway collapse. These smooth-muscle fibers are reduced in HDAC patients; this is in contrast to the reduction in cartilaginous structures noted in TBM.[1,2]

Lastly, the impaired mucociliary clearance and recurrent respiratory infections in many TBM/HDAC patients often results in inflammation, contributing to further airway damage.[1,2]

ETIOLOGY

TBM and HDAC may be congenital (primary) or acquired (secondary). Nearly all congenital cases are due to genetic diseases that weaken the trachea and present during childhood (eg, mucopolychondritis). One congenital tracheomegaly that usually presents in adulthood is idiopathic giant trachea (IGT), which occurs as a result of atrophy of longitudinal elastic fibers and muscularis mucosa.[9] When this atrophy perpetuates into the central bronchi, it can result in congenital tracheobronchomegaly, also known as Mounier-Kuhn syndrome.[9] Adult TBM and HDAC can also be caused by Ehlers-Danlos syndrome, an inherited collagen-vascular disease associated with weakening or laxity of cartilaginous structures.[2] Nevertheless, the vast majority of adult cases of TBM and HDAC are acquired, and these form the focus of this discussion (**Box 1**). Airway inflammation and/or mechanical manipulation of the airway are the most common secondary causes of adult acquired TBM and HDAC. An accurate history and physical examination combined with a careful review of the patient's diagnostic information will likely identify the source of the problem.

There is a myriad of causes of chronic or acute airway inflammation associated with TBM and HDAC. First, irritants may be inhaled or aspirated into the airways. Among inhalants, fossil-fuel consumption by-products and tobacco smoke have both been implicated, as have toxins such as mustard gas.[2,10] Aspirated materials, such as food or gastric acid, can also cause airway damage. Second, recurrent airway infections can result in severe chronic airway inflammation; therefore, cystic fibrosis and immunodeficiencies can both lead to TBM and HDAC.[1,2,6] Third, common pulmonary diseases such as asthma and chronic obstructive pulmonary disease (COPD) may also cause TBM and HDAC owing to chronic inflammation of the airway wall, not to mention changes in chest pressure that may precipitate collapse of large airways.[1,2] Finally, collagen-vascular diseases such as relapsing polychondritis can also be causative.[1,2,11]

Among mechanical causes of TBM and HDAC, generally either some form of airway manipulation/mechanical injury or chronic external tracheal compression is responsible.[1,2] Posttraumatic causes include closed-chest trauma (which can lead to tracheal cartilage fracture and airway-wall weakening), surgeries (eg, lung transplantation), endobronchial electrosurgery, laser therapy, tracheostomy, or endotracheal intubation (particularly if prolonged).[12] Chronic external compression of the trachea can result from nonmalignant masses (such as benign mediastinal goiter, aortic or pulmonary artery aneurysm, cysts, abscesses, vascular rings, or even obesity).

Box 1
Etiology of TBM and HDAC

- Airway inflammation
  - Irritant inhalation/aspiration
    - Inhalation of chemical irritants (eg, tobacco smoke, fossil-fuel combustion by-products)
    - Aspiration/gastroesophageal reflux disease
  - Recurrent airway infections (as can be seen in cystic fibrosis, primary ciliary dyskinesias, bronchiectasis, and immunodeficiencies)
  - Common pulmonary diseases (eg, chronic obstructive pulmonary disease, asthma)
  - Collagen vascular diseases (eg, relapsing polychondritis)
  - Prolonged intubation
  - Tracheostomy
- Mechanical causes
  - Injury or manipulation of the airway
    - Closed-chest trauma
    - Tracheal surgery (lung resection, lung transplant)
    - Tracheostomy
    - Endotracheal or endobronchial electrosurgery or laser therapy
  - Chronic external tracheal compression
    - Airway or lung malignancy
    - Nonmalignant chest anomalies (eg, thyroid goiter, aortic or pulmonary artery aneurysm, bronchogenic cysts, abscesses, vascular rings, obesity)
- Congenital diseases presenting in adulthood
  - Mounier-Kuhn syndrome (congenital tracheobronchomegaly)
  - Ehlers-Danlos syndrome

Malignancies of the airways or lungs can cause TBM and HDAC by either mechanical compression or destruction of tissue itself.

CLASSIFICATION

The classification of TBM and HDAC is more than academic; it carries significant ramifications for decisions regarding appropriate treatment. TBM and HDAC can be classified based on location (proximal vs distal), distribution (segmental or diffuse), type of airway luminal narrowing (tracheal appearance), severity (mild, moderate, or severe), or etiology (congenital or acquired; see previous section).[3]

Location is an important determinant of treatment, as only proximal TBM and HDAC (involving the trachea, proximal mainstem bronchi, or both) is an appropriate candidate for invasive measures such as airway stenting and surgical repair. Distal TBM and HDAC can only be managed medically. Distribution may also have some impact on treatment decisions, as diffuse disease may be more difficult than segmental disease for stenting, surgery, or laser application.[2]

Tracheal appearance is another way to classify TBM and HDAC, and it may assist in identifying the cause of a patient's disease. Lateral tracheal narrowing (saber-sheath or fissure shaped) is usually due to COPD.[2] Anteroposterior tracheal flattening (crescent or scabbard shaped) or concentric narrowing is associated with relapsing polychondritis (**Fig. 1**).[11]

Severity of TBM and HDAC may determine therapeutic decisions. Airway narrowing that is mild (lumen reduction of 50%–70%) or moderate (lumen reduction of 70%–90%) is generally managed medically, with treatment of the underlying cause being paramount. Severe disease (lumen reduction greater than 90%), if accompanied by severe symptoms, should be evaluated for stenting and surgical repair.[1,2] Nevertheless, as in patients with less severe disease, any primary contributing cause should still be aggressively targeted.

CLINICAL MANIFESTATIONS

The clinical presentation of TBM and HDAC is nonspecific and mimics other conditions, making a constant level of awareness important (**Box 2**). If airway compromise

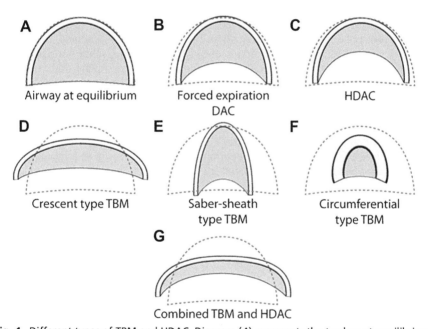

Fig. 1. Different types of TBM and HDAC. Diagram (*A*) represents the trachea at equilibrium, with the posterior membrane being flat. In (*B*) through (*F*), the dotted line represents the trachea at equilibrium, with the solid lines representing changes with forced expiration. (*B*) represents forced exhalation in the normal individual; note how the posterior membrane bulges forward into the lumen of the airway. (*C*) represents forced exhalation in HDAC, with the posterior membrane bulging into the lumen of the airway and occluding more than 50% of the airway lumen. Note that the integrity of the tracheal ring is intact in shape and configuration. (*D*) represents crescent-type TBM that manifests with flattening of the tracheal cartilaginous rings, and is evidence of loss of structural integrity. Note that the membranous portion of the trachea is flat and not bulging into the lumen of the airway. The main site of abnormality is in the tracheal cartilage. (*E*) represents saber-sheath type TBM and manifests with inward movement of the lateral walls. It is commonly seen in patients with chronic obstructive pulmonary disease. (*F*) represents concentric TBM with both anterior and lateral wall movement. It is typically seen with severe airway-wall inflammation. (*G*) represents combined TBM and HDAC. In this combined form the cartilaginous structures flatten, and the posterior membrane bulges into the airway lumen. This form is the one most commonly encountered in the adult population.

Box 2
Signs and symptoms of TBM and HDAC

Dyspnea

Intractable cough (often barking)

Recurrent pulmonary infections (eg, bronchitis, pneumonias)

Difficulty expectorating sputum

Wheezing/stridor

Hemoptysis

Syncope due to cough

---

is mild, patients may be asymptomatic. Major signs and symptoms include dyspnea, intractable cough (occasionally with severe paroxysms), and impaired clearance of secretions. In turn, this impaired mucociliary clearance results in sputum retention and recurrent pulmonary infections such as bronchitis and pneumonias.[1,2] Patients with TBM and HDAC will often complain of dyspnea and cough that are particularly exacerbated with exercise. In addition, patients frequently complain that complete exhalation is difficult; inhalation is typically not troublesome.

The signs and symptoms of TBM and HDAC are nonspecific. If patients fail to respond to the usual and customary treatment of a suspected respiratory condition, consideration should be given to evaluation for TBM and HDAC. Signs and symptoms may include wheezing/stridor, barking cough, episodic choking, syncope associated with forced exhalation/cough, and recurrent pulmonary infections (bronchitis and pneumonias caused by impaired mucociliary clearance).[13–15]

Aside from exercise, other maneuvers that may elicit signs and symptoms are Valsalva maneuvers, positional changes (particularly recumbency), and forced exhalation/cough.

Because these signs and symptoms may be present in many other conditions, it is critical to maintain a level of suspicion when a clinical presentation for a presumed diagnosis is atypical. Such a situation may involve symptoms that are disproportionate to other known conditions (eg, asthma, COPD) or a failure to respond to typical treatment modalities.

DIFFERENTIAL DIAGNOSIS

As already noted, the signs and symptoms of TBM and HDAC are nonspecific, and may mimic many diseases. The broad differential diagnosis includes asthma, COPD (both emphysema and chronic bronchitis), and cigarette smoking. Other conditions that could cause at least some of the typical signs and symptoms are cardiac disease (such as congestive heart failure), bronchiectasis, immunodeficiency, cystic fibrosis, primary ciliary dyskinesias, obesity hypoventilation syndrome, chronic gastroesophageal reflux disease (GERD), and recurrent aspiration.

DIAGNOSIS

The diagnostic approach to TBM and HDAC follows a fairly uniform algorithm once it is suspected (**Table 1**). Evaluation is usually begun based on initial history with suggestive symptoms/signs (such as symptoms disproportionate to a given diagnosis or failure to respond to standard treatment), or suspected after pulmonary function testing or chest radiography. The 2 initial diagnostic evaluations that should be

Table 1
Diagnostic testing for TBM and HDAC

Test	Findings: TBM and HDAC	Importance
Pulmonary function testing	Diminished expiratory flow Abnormal flow volume loop Notching of expiratory flow loop	Identify respiratory functional impact; rule out concomitant asthma and emphysema
Computed tomography of the chest with dynamic expiratory imaging	Narrowing of airway lumen with expiratory maneuver	Identify the severity of airway narrowing. Potentially identify specific etiologic factors responsible for TBM or HDAC and thereby direct specific management. Rule out alternative causes of patient's complaints
Bronchoscopy with forced expiratory maneuvers	Narrowing of airway lumen with expiratory maneuver	Identify severity of airway narrowing. May biopsy tracheal wall or collect culture specimens
pH or impedance-probe testing	Active reflux to the proximal aerodigestive tract	Reducing or stopping active reflux may alleviate symptoms associated with TBM and HDAC and stabilize the airway

Pulmonary function testing should be completed in all patients being evaluated for TBM or HDAC. Respiratory diseases often coexist or cause TBM and HDAC. Proper recognition as well as aggressive therapy is indicated in patients with specific respiratory diagnoses. Computed tomography (CT) of the chest with dynamic expiratory imaging is a valuable test. Chest CT may also identify a specific source that is causing complaints and offer therapeutic guidance. Bronchoscopy with airway examination is considered the gold standard for diagnosing TBM and HDAC. Bronchoscopy allows location of the TBM or HDAC and gradation of the severity of collapse, while providing an opportunity to sample the affected tissue or collect culture specimens (if a chronic infection is suspected). Nasogastric pH or impedance-probe testing can solidify the diagnosis of aspiration and reflux of gastric contents in patients who are suspected of having reflux-related airway involvement. A polysomnogram should be obtained in patients who have signs and symptoms of sleep apnea. Finally, serologies may be considered in patients who are suspected of having collagen vascular disease, as they may identify a possible therapeutic target.

performed in all patients with suspected TBM and HDAC are pulmonary function tests and computed tomography (CT) of the chest with dynamic expiratory imaging. The diagnostic standard is bronchoscopy; other tests may be performed depending on the clinical circumstances.

Pulmonary function tests primarily help in ruling out severe obstructive or restrictive lung disease as the primary cause of symptoms. Often, obstructive lung disease leads to HDAC rather than TBM. It is almost impossible to differentiate COPD from TBM/HDAC as a main cause of symptoms by pulmonary function testing alone. A dynamic CT of the chest can help differentiate patients with and without TBM/HDAC. If TBM/HDAC is significant and symptoms of dyspnea on exertion are out of proportion to a patient's COPD, a stent trial should be considered.[2] The flow-volume loop can show a low peak expiratory flow rate, with a subsequent rapid decrease in flow rate. Garcia-Pachon[16] found that 1.4% of subjects had expiratory flow-volume loops with flow oscillations (alternating accelerations and decelerations of flow); physiologic upper airway obstruction was also noted in 35% of this population.

Chest CT with dynamic expiratory imaging is invaluable in the diagnosis of TBM and HDAC. This procedure involves having the patient perform a forced exhalation and then capturing end-expiratory images to measure a cross section of the trachea and bronchi.[1,2] CT imaging can aid in determining if TBM and HDAC are present, and can indicate a possible cause. Accuracy in some studies was up to 97%; on the other hand, in another study up to 78% of normal patients had 50% luminal narrowing.[4,17–20]

Bronchoscopy is acknowledged to be the gold-standard diagnostic measure for TBM and HDAC, and should be performed in all patients with a strong suspicion for this disease.[1] Bronchoscopy can identify the presence of airway narrowing, assess its severity, and classify its distribution and location. If indicated, endobronchial biopsies may be obtained as well. The primary advantage of bronchoscopy is direct visualization in real time of the trachea and bronchi during forced exhalations and tidal breathing. Therefore, it is imperative that patients not be excessively sedated, as this will impair maximum exhalation efforts and the ability to follow commands. Some studies have used other maneuvers during bronchoscopy, such as coughing. However, eliciting coughing can cause near or complete airway collapse in even normal patients and therefore is not recommended. In regards to determination of future therapy, bronchoscopy helps by revealing ease of airway navigation. On the other hand, CT is superior for visualizing TBM distal extension into segmental and subsegmental bronchi (neither of which can be corrected by stenting or surgery).[3]

Finally, a 24-hour impedance/pH probe study is advised if GERD is suspected (either because of patients' complaints or suggestive imaging). If acid or nonacid reflux is present, effective treatment may stop the airway inflammatory process and reverse TBM and HDAC.[21]

TREATMENT

The treatment algorithm for TBM and HDAC involves first determining symptoms and severity. If a patient is asymptomatic, treatment is unnecessary even when objective disease is severe. If respiratory symptoms are disproportionate to an individual's mild TBM and HDAC, investigation for other factors should be performed. If a patient has evidence of moderate to severe TBM and HDAC and signs and symptoms correlate, appropriate treatment of this condition is indicated.

The second component of treatment involves medical management of underlying causes and comorbid conditions.[1,2] Such management may even suffice to cause cessation of symptoms, particularly in cases where severe recurrent infections or severe aspiration are the primary causes.[1,2,11] If GERD and aspiration cannot be controlled medically, surgical intervention such as Nissen fundoplication may be necessary.[21] Other causes of chronic airway inflammation similarly need to be addressed. Aggressive immune suppression can be used for collagen-vascular diseases such as relapsing polychondritis. If there is concomitant asthma or COPD, maximum treatment is indicated.[1,2] Appropriate breathing techniques and exercise programs also may provide ancillary benefits. Obstructive sleep apnea should be treated with noninvasive positive pressure ventilation (NIPPV); NIPPV pneumatically stents the airway, which may in turn improve airway clearance and reduce inflammation.[2,22]

A critical component of the treatment of TBM and HDAC is aggressive weight management. Obesity results in several anatomic changes, including diaphragm elevation and downward movement of the chest wall, both of which result in foreshortening and reduced rigidity of the trachea. These changes can be reversed by weight loss, potentially resolving TBM and HDAC. Treatment of obesity and other potential contributing factors is crucial for therapeutic success, as long-term surgical outcomes are significantly poorer if these factors are not adequately treated.

If symptoms persist despite aggressive medical management of underlying causes and comorbid conditions, stent trialing and surgical correction need to be considered. Before this, functional status should be evaluated to determine a baseline for comparison with objective evaluations in the future. In addition to pulmonary function testing as already described, this should include a 6-minute walk test and quality-of-life assessment.[1]

A stent trial is indicated for nearly all TBM and HDAC patients before surgery.[23] One possible exception is when the predominant symptom is not dyspnea, but instead paroxysmal cough or recurrent infections. In this case, determination for surgery may need to be based on abnormal anatomy alone, as stenting may not help.[3] If a patient objectively improves and is a surgical candidate, the next step is to evaluate for definitive surgical correction. However, if a patient fails to objectively improve with a stent trial, surgical repair is not typically indicated, and a therapeutic trial of NIPPV should be considered instead. In general, long-term airway stenting is not recommended; complications may result, such as inspissation of secretions leading to stent blockage and granulation.[24] Patients who are not considered surgical candidates should therefore generally not receive stent trials in the first place.

The details of airway stents are beyond the scope of this review, but the general principles are as follows. There are 2 main types of stents, silicone and metal. Metal stents, though useful in other forms of airway obstruction, are suboptimal for TBM and HDAC because of frequent complications and difficulty of removal.[1] Instead, silicone stents, typically in the shape of an inverted "Y" because of the low chance of migration, are the modality of choice. These stents are placed by a rigid bronchoscope under general anesthesia. In many studies,[23] stenting resulted in immediate airflow and symptom improvement; a usual time period for a stent trial is about 2 weeks. Repeat objective evaluation such as pulmonary function testing, 6-minute walk test, and quality-of-life assessment should be performed.

The definitive surgical treatment of choice for TBM and HDAC is tracheobronchoplasty, which entails suturing a polypropylene mesh to the posterior tracheal membrane, thereby increasing the airway's rigidity (**Fig. 2**).[23] A lengthy procedure, it requires a right posterolateral thoracotomy approach to access the bilateral bronchi and thoracic trachea. Appropriate selection of patients, surgeons, and treatment centers is important. In the United States there are only a handful of physicians and treatment centers with a good deal of experience in tracheobronchoplasty. Patient selection is equally critical, but Majid and colleagues[23] found that in comparison with baseline, it significantly improved multiple end points: dyspnea, quality of life, mean exercise capacity, and functional status.

As noted earlier, NIPPV in the form of continuous positive airway pressure (CPAP) can improve TBM and HDAC by maintaining an open airway and aiding in drainage of secretions. It has been found that during acute illnesses it is useful to initiate continuous CPAP, followed by intermittent CPAP as symptoms improve.[3] Unfortunately, it has not been shown to improve dyspnea or coughing over the long term.[25] CPAP is generally used; however, bilevel airway pressure may be used instead if there is hypercapnic respiratory failure.[3]

In cases of focal HDAC, topical laser application therapy has been useful.[2] A laser is applied to membranous portions of the patient's trachea or bronchi, creating scarring that contracts and stiffens the posterior membrane.[2,26]

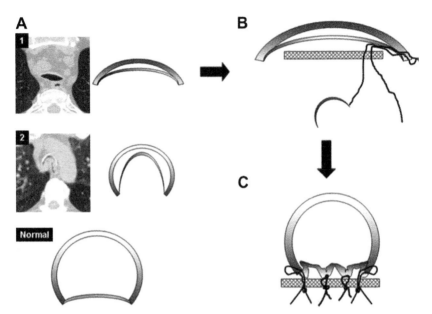

Fig. 2. Malacic airway abnormality in cross section and correction with tracheobroncho-plasty. (*A*) Airway (1) represents the form of TBM that primarily affects the cartilage, causing lateral migration of the cartilaginous-membranous junction and decreased ratio of sagittal/coronal diameter. A representative CT image accompanies the diagram. Airway (2) represents the form of TBM that primarily is manifest by intrusion of the membranous wall into the lumen of the airway, with relative preservation of coronal diameter. A representative CT image accompanies the diagram. A normal airway cross section (Normal) is also depicted. (*B*) Posterior splinting. Mesh is represented by the cross-hatched rectangle, and suture is seen passed in partial-thickness, mattressed fashion through the airway wall. (*C*) After sutures are tied down, any redundancy of the membranous wall is pleated to the mesh, and the D-shape of the airway is restored. (*Reprinted from* Gangadharan SP. Tracheobronchomalacia in adults. Semin Thoracic Surg 2010;22:165–73; with permission from Elsevier Inc.)

In the future, treatment might include tracheal replacement or biogenic stents. Tracheal replacement would involve placement of a new trachea to replace the defective trachea. Biogenic stents, which gradually integrate into the airway wall, would have the advantage of minimally invasive placement. These stents could also potentially maintain normal mucociliary clearance while preventing airway collapse.

SUMMARY

TBM and HDAC are distinct diseases with significant clinical overlap. TBM involves loss of structural integrity of the cartilaginous structures of the airway wall, whereas HDAC is exaggeration of normal airway-wall movement with luminal intrusion of the posterior membrane. Nevertheless, both result in airway compromise. Signs and symptoms include dyspnea and cough worsened with exercise, as well as poor mucociliary clearance. TBM and HDAC can mimic asthma and should be suspected in individuals with symptoms disproportionate to an initial diagnosis, or in patients who fail to respond to appropriate treatment for this diagnosis. Diagnostic evaluation includes chest CT with dynamic expiratory imaging, pulmonary function tests, and the gold standard of bronchoscopy. Treatment includes aggressive medical management of contributing causes (whether inflammatory or mechanical) and comorbid conditions. If symptoms persist, a trial of airway stenting is indicated to identify individuals who should receive definitive surgical correction with tracheobronchoplasty.

REFERENCES

1. Carden KA, Boiselle PM, Waltz DA, et al. Tracheomalacia and tracheobroncho-malacia in children and adults: an in-depth review. Chest 2005;127:984–1005.
2. Murgu SD, Colt HG. Tracheobronchomalacia and excessive dynamic airway collapse. Respirology 2006;11:388–406.
3. Ernst A, Carden K, Gangadharan SP. Tracheomalacia and tracheobronchomala-cia in adults. UpToDate.com [Internet]. Updated 2012 Jul 9. Available at: http://www.uptodate.com/contents/tracheomalacia-and-tracheobronchomalacia-in-adults. Accessed on October 4th, 2012.
4. Boiselle PM, O'Donnell CR, Bankier AA, et al. Tracheal collapsibility in healthy volunteers during forced expiration: assessment with multidetector CT. Radiology 2009;252:255–62.
5. Ochs RA, Petkovska I, Kim HJ, et al. Prevalence of tracheal collapse in an emphysema cohort measured with end-expiration CT. Acad Radiol 2009;16: 46–53.
6. Jokinen K, Palva T, Sutinen S, et al. Acquired tracheobronchomalacia. Ann Clin Res 1977;9:52–7.
7. Hasegawa I, Boiselle PM, Raptopoulos V, et al. Tracheomalacia incidentally detected on CT pulmonary angiography of patients with suspected pulmonary embolism. AJR Am J Roentgenol 2003;181:1505–9.
8. Nuutinen J. Acquired tracheobronchomalacia. A clinical study with bronchologi-cal correlations. Ann Clin Res 1977;9:350.
9. Schwartz M, Rossoff L. Tracheobronchomegaly—Mounier-Kuhn syndrome. Br J Radiol 1984;57:640.
10. Ghanei M, Akbari Moqadam F, Mohammad MM, et al. Tracheobronchomalacia and air trapping after mustard gas exposure. Am J Respir Crit Care Med 2006; 173:304.
11. Ernst A, Rafeq S, Boiselle P, et al. Relapsing polychondritis and airway involve-ment. Chest 2009;135:1024–30.
12. Norwood S, Vallina VL, Short K, et al. Incidence of tracheal stenosis and other late complications after percutaneous tracheostomy. Ann Surg 2000;232:233–41.
13. Nuutinen J. Acquired tracheobronchomalacia. A bronchological follow-up study. Ann Clin Res 1977;9:359.
14. Johnson TH, Mikita JJ, Wilson RJ, et al. Acquired tracheomalacia. Radiology 1973;109:576.
15. Imaizumi H, Kaneko M, Mori K, et al. Reversible acquired tracheobronchomalacia of a combined crescent type and saber-sheath type. J Emerg Med 1995;13:43.
16. Garcia-Pachon E. Tracheobronchomalacia: a cause of flow oscillations on the flow-volume loop. Chest 2000;118:1519.
17. Gilkeson RC, Ciancibello LM, Hejal RB, et al. Tracheobronchomalacia: dynamic airway evaluation with multidetector CT. AJR Am J Roentgenol 2001;176:205.
18. Aquino SL, Shepard JA, Ginns LC, et al. Acquired tracheomalacia: detection by expiratory CT scan. J Comput Assist Tomogr 2001;25:394.
19. Stern EJ, Graham CM, Webb WR, et al. Normal trachea during forced expiration: dynamic CT measurements. Radiology 1993;187:27.

20. Lee KS, Sun MR, Ernst A, et al. Comparison of dynamic expiratory CT with bronchoscopy for diagnosing airway malacia: a pilot evaluation. Chest 2007;131:758.
21. Kovesi T, Rubin S. Long-term complications of congenital esophageal atresia and/or tracheoesophageal fistula. Chest 2004;126:915–25.
22. Adliff M, Ngato D, Keshavjee S, et al. Treatment of diffuse tracheomalacia secondary to relapsing polychondritis with continuous positive airway pressure. Chest 1997;112:1701–4.
23. Majid A, Guerrero J, Gangadharan S, et al. Tracheobronchoplasty for severe tracheobronchomalacia: a prospective outcome analysis. Chest 2008;134:801–7.
24. Ernst A, Majid A, Feller-Kopman D, et al. Airway stabilization with silicone stents for treating adult tracheobronchomalacia: a prospective observational study. Chest 2007;132:609–16.
25. Ferguson GT, Benoist J. Nasal continuous positive airway pressure in the treatment of tracheobronchomalacia. Am Rev Respir Dis 1993;147:457.
26. Dutau H, Breen DP. Endobronchial laser treatment: an essential tool in therapeutic bronchoscopy. Eur Respir Mon 2010;48:149–60.

Cardiac Asthma

Kern Buckner, MD

KEYWORDS

- Dyspnea • Asthma • Congestive heart failure • Cardiomyopathy
- Pulmonary venous hypertension

KEY POINTS

- Cardiac dyspnea, especially if present only with exercise, is often confused with asthma and exercise-induced bronchospasm.
- Cardiac asthma is the consequence of pulmonary edema due to pulmonary venous hypertension and not due to asthmatic bronchoconstriction.
- In overt, acute congestive heart failure, the diagnosis may be readily made by history and physical examination and pertinent laboratory and imaging data but other more subtle, or compensated, presentations of heart failure, especially diastolic dysfunction, may present a diagnostic challenge to the bedside clinician.
- In distinguishing cardiac from pulmonary dyspnea, the most useful and informative studies include a serum B-type natriuretic peptide, an echocardiogram, and if necessary, a cardiopulmonary stress test.

DEFINITION

Simply put, cardiac asthma applies to breathing difficulties due to cardiogenic pulmonary edema. The pathogenesis is not asthmatic bronchoconstriction but rather a reflex bronchoconstriction as a manifestation of pulmonary congestion due to pulmonary venous hypertension (PVH). Cardiac dyspnea may be a more appropriate broader definition. Cardiac asthma is but one presentation of cardiac dyspnea.

Heart failure can be defined as systolic failure with a reduced left ventricular ejection fraction (HFrEF) or diastolic dysfunction due to a stiff heart or valvular heart disease, but with a preserved left ventricular ejection fraction (HFpEF). Heart failure has also been classified as right or left-sided. Cardiac dyspnea due to PVH represents left-sided failure that manifests as pulmonary congestion. For the purposes of the author's discussion, heart failure will represent left-sided heart failure.

HISTORY OF CARDIAC ASTHMA

The understanding that lung ailments may be of cardiac origin has dated back to antiquity.[1] The first reference to "cardiac asthma" was in 1833 when James Hope

Division of Cardiology, Department of Medicine, National Jewish Health, 1400 Jackson Street, Denver, CO 80206, USA
E-mail address: bucknerk@njhealth.org

Immunol Allergy Clin N Am 33 (2013) 35–44
http://dx.doi.org/10.1016/j.iac.2012.10.012
0889-8561/13/$ – see front matter © 2013 Elsevier Inc. All rights reserved.

coined the term, and by 1854, cardiac asthma was considered a disease state.[1] Sir William Osler's classic description in 1897 remains as true today as then. "In the case of advanced arteriosclerosis, there are often attacks of dyspnea of great intensity recurring in paroxysms, often nocturnal. The patient goes to bed feeling quite well, and in the early morning hours wakes in an attack which, in its abruptness of onset and general features, resembles asthma. Two other features about this form of attack will attract your attention...the evident effort in breathing and the presence of a wheezing in the bronchial tubes, and of moist rales at the base of the lungs."[1,2] Although cardiac asthma has been historically considered a hallmark of congestive heart disease, today's understanding of exercise physiology and diastolic dysfunction broaden the definition to any pathologic cardiac condition that is exacerbated with increased venous return.

The initial descriptions of cardiac asthma were reported in patients with late stage systolic failure (HFrEF), usually due to ischemic or hypertensive cardiomyopathy or mitral stenosis from rheumatic mitral valve disease (HFpEF). These cases were also described in lesser stages of heart failure with provocation of congestion due to the increased metabolic demands and increased venous return of strenuous exercise.

The allergy/immunology or pulmonology physician is often faced with the challenge of deciding if dyspnea is of pulmonary (e.g., asthma) or cardiac origin. The understanding of the mechanisms and manifestations of cardiac dyspnea will be useful in distinguishing cardiac from pulmonary dyspnea.

PATHOPHYSIOLOGY

The pathophysiology of congestive heart failure is manifested in the lung as the consequence of PVH. A good understanding of PVH and its effects on the mechanical and gas exchange properties of the lungs is necessary to effectively distinguish cardiac from pulmonary dyspnea.

Under normal, resting, and upright conditions, pulmonary blood flow is influenced by the impact of gravity, resulting in an incremental, linear increase of blood flow to bases compared with the apices of the lung.

Left atrial hypertension develops as a consequence of left ventricular dysfunction. Elevated left atrial pressures, in turn, create PVH to preserve a negative flow gradient. PVH reduces the gravitational pressure gradient and more evenly distributes pulmonary blood flow by distention and recruitment of pulmonary capillaries.[3–5]

The clinical manifestations of PVH are variable and influenced by its time course (acute or chronic) and severity. Initially, with modest increases in pulmonary venous pressure, the recruitment and distension of the lung capillary bed mitigates the pressure difference and protects the capillary bed from pulmonary edema.

The flux of water across the capillary is regulated at the capillary microvascular barrier by the opposing forces of capillary hydrostatic pressure and the interstitial oncotic pressure. The anatomic structure of the alveolar-capillary unit favors gas exchange and protects from increased hydrostatic pressure by encouraging edema formation in the interstitial compartment.[6] With increasing hydrostatic pressure, intravascular fluid transudates from the capillary to the interstitium across an oncotic gradient and mitigates the tendency of increased hydrostatic pressure to cause pulmonary edema.[6] In doing so, gas exchange is protected.

Fluid in the interstitium is rapidly transported by negative pressure gradient to the hilum and the pleural space.[7] Lymphatic vessels within these tissues are able to clear large volumes of lung water.[7,8]

Chronic elevated hydrostatic pressure ultimately leads to the disruption of the protective layers of the alveolar-capillary unit. The disrupted integrity of the capillary membrane allows proteins and water to flux across the capillary bed into the alveolar sac as pulmonary edema.[9,10]

PVH and increased hydrostatic pressures within the capillary promote precapillary vascular changes. In response to the increased capillary pressure, there is remodeling of the precapillary arterioles, initially with an increase in vascular tone, including medial hypertrophy from "muscularization." For reasons not well understood, vascular remodeling may progress to intimal and adventitial hyperplasia and plexiform lesions, and the development of obstructive vasculopathy. The progression of vascular remodeling is associated with increased pulmonary vascular resistance. The increased vascular tone may be reversible, but the hyperplastic remodeling appears to not be reversible and portends a poor prognosis.

Pulmonary function is greatly influenced by lung water. Excess lung water can produce a loss of total lung capacity from multiple mechanisms, including displacement of lung from an enlarged heart, interstitial edema, loss of lung compliance, pleural effusions, and increased work of breathing leading to respiratory muscle fatigue.[11] Airway resistance may be increased and wheezing auscultated, but airflow obstruction is uncommon.[12] Several mechanisms have been postulated for the increased airway resistance and wheezing: (1) elevation of capillary hydrostatic pressure and edema causing reflex bronchoconstriction; (2) reduced geometric bronchial size due to reduced lung volumes; (3) bronchial obstruction from intraluminal edema; and (4) bronchial mucosal edema.[13] Normalization of pulmonary function has been reported in appropriately treated mitral valve disease or nonvalvular congestive heart failure, including post-mitral valve replacement or post-heart transplantation.[14,15]

CLINICAL PRESENTATION
History

The clinical presentation of cardiac asthma has been classically described as nocturnal dyspnea in the recumbent position. After 2 to 4 hours of sleep, the patient awakens with a start and the sensation of smothering or impending doom, unable to get an adequate breath, and quickly has to sit on the side of the bed or go to the window for fresh air. The patient may experience an audible wheeze or a cough; this cough may be dry or productive of minimal mucus, but on occasion may be associated with blood-tinged sputum. On sitting or standing for several minutes, the attack subsides, and the patient returns to bed to sleep throughout the remainder of the night.

The history mentioned earlier typifies a patient who has marginally compensated congestive heart failure during the waking hours but decompensates at night due to the increase in venous return associated with the recumbent position. This often represents later stage heart failure, and the diagnosis is confirmed with minimal further investigation of physical examination and ancillary studies.

Other, more subtle presentations of congestive heart failure may represent a diagnostic challenge to the bedside clinician. Chronic heart failure that is well compensated may often elude even the most thorough history unless a prior history of heart disease is obtained.

Heart failure is defined as the inability of cardiac function to meet the metabolic demands of the body. Heart failure presentations are usually heralded by the symptoms of congestion, of low cardiac output, or a combination of both. Although heart failure affects the global integrated right and left heart function, the concept has been traditionally categorized by considering the individual right and left heart pumps. Keeping in mind that the most common cause of right heart failure is left heart failure, and the greater prevalence of left heart disease than isolated right heart disease, approaching the evaluation of heart failure from a left ventricular bias offers an excellent initial approach.

The cardinal symptoms of heart failure are dyspnea, fatigue, and exertional intolerance. Early in heart disease and failure, dyspnea is only provoked with exertion. However, as heart disease advances, the dyspnea occurs with less and less activity. In the latter stages of heart failure, dyspnea progresses to orthopnea, and paroxysmal dyspnea may be present.

Symptoms of cardiac congestion may be either left sided or right sided or a combination of both. Left heart congestion is manifested as pulmonary edema and characterized by varying degrees of dyspnea. The *sine qua non* of left heart failure is orthopnea and paroxysmal nocturnal dyspnea, reflecting the left heart's inability to compensate for the increased venous return due to the recumbent position. The defining symptoms of right heart failure are systemic edema of the lower extremities or ascites and reflect gravitational dependency and elevated right heart pressures.

Low cardiac output may be of either right or left heart origin, and symptoms are usually expressed as fatigue, mental status alteration, and the periodic respiration of Cheyne-Stokes. Orthostatic intolerance may be present in the latter stages of heart failure or with the use of vasoactive medications, and is aggravated if the patient is overdiuresed.

In the later stages of heart failure, functional class III or IV (**Table 1**), symptoms of dyspnea and fatigue, orthopnea and paroxysmal nocturnal dyspnea, and lower extremity edema or ascites may be easy to elicit and readily establish the presence of a failing heart. Patients with chronic obstructive pulmonary disease (COPD) may also complain of similar symptoms due to breathing mechanics that require a more upright position. The sputum expectoration of COPD may help to distinguish the cause.

The earlier stages of heart disease, functional class I and II (see **Table 1**), may be challenging to diagnose. Symptoms, (typically dyspnea), are often only experienced with the increased metabolic demands and venous return of exertion or exercise. These latter, less symptomatic classifications of heart disease require a careful history to raise the suspicion of cardiac dyspnea. Herein lies the diagnostic dilemma of cardiac versus pulmonary origin of dyspnea (see **Table 1**).

Dyspnea is the sentinel symptom of heart disease, and its onset, timing, and severity correlates with the extent of cardiac dysfunction. As with other disease states in the body, the demands of exertion may unmask underlying but adequately compensated heart disease. In the early stages of some heart disease, symptoms of dyspnea may be subtle and hard to quantitate and require the objective assessment of a stress test, preferably a cardiopulmonary exercise tolerance test, if available.

History should include an assessment of prior heart disease or risk factors for developing cardiac dyspnea or heart failure. This identifies a patient population likely to have an element of cardiac dyspnea. Diagnoses such as angina or prior myocardial infarction or mechanical coronary revascularization, hypertension, valvular heart

Table 1 New York Heart Association classification system	
Class I	No symptoms with ordinary activity: no limitation to physical activity
Class II	Symptoms with ordinary activity: mild limitation of physical activity
Class III	Symptoms with less than ordinary activity: marked limitation of physical activity
Class IV	Symptoms at rest: severe limitation of physical activity

Data from Criteria Committee, New York Heart Association. Diseases of the heart and blood vessels: nomenclature and criteria for diagnosis. 6th edition. Boston: Little, Brown; 1964.

disease, or diabetes, to name some of the more common risk factors, should be cataloged and investigated for stability and compensation.

Even in absence of the patients' understanding of their underlying disease process, a medication list that includes a diuretic, β-blocker, angiotensin-converting enzyme (ACE) inhibitor, angiotensin receptor blocker, antiarrhythmic agent, or calcium channel blocker should alert the physician to the probability of heart disease. Inquiry should be made regarding those conditions such as anemia, hypoxia, tachycardia, thyroid dysfunction, medication noncompliance, or renal insufficiency that may decompensate underlying heart disease. Commonly used nonsteroidal antiinflammatory drugs alter prostaglandin sensitive renal blood flow and may lead to salt and fluid retention and exacerbate congestive heart failure. The glitazones (e.g., pioglitazone and rosiglitazone) also cause fluid retention and may be responsible for an exacerbation of heart failure.

Physical Examination

The history should prompt a more focused examination for either the presence of heart failure or those conditions that predispose to heart failure. In many cases, the physical examination can confirm the diagnosis of congestive heart failure and explain the cause of dyspnea. However, in many cases the resting heart examination will be normal; this does not exclude heart disease without other confirmatory laboratory or imaging data.

The physical examination should also key on assessing the physical manifestations of congestion and low cardiac output. These findings may not be present in the early stages of heart failure, and the pulmonary findings may be diminished or absent in chronic, compensated heart failure (even in the latter stages of heart failure) or in the comorbid condition of COPD, especially emphysema.[16,17]

The constellation of an apical S3 or summation gallop, basilar rales, basilar dullness to percussion, elevated jugular vein distention (JVD), and pretibial edema should alert the physician to left heart failure and associated right heart failure. On occasion, the rales are accompanied by expiratory squeaks or wheezes and termed "cardiac asthma." In chronic left heart failure, the recruitment of extensive lymphatic drainage in the lungs may clear the excessive fluid accumulation. In these circumstances, rales may not be auscultated despite pulmonary wedge pressures in excess of 20 mm Hg. In patients with coexisting emphysema, rales may be masked by the overall reduction in breath sounds. Hepatojugular reflux (HJR) may unmask occult right heart failure that is otherwise compensated. Hepatomegaly or a pulsatile liver, with or without ascites, in the context of JVD or HJR establishes cardiac heart failure. COPD with hyperinflatation of the lungs may displace the liver and mimic hepatomegaly.[16]

The physical signs of low cardiac output reflect insufficient perfusion. Abnormal cardiac pulses such as pulsus alternans (left ventricular ejection fraction <30%) or narrow pulse pressure reflect left ventricular systolic dysfunction and low cardiac output state. Cool extremities, lethargy, or mental obtundation are signs of decreased cardiac perfusion.

Structural heart disease may present as a mumur, gallop, or abnormal point of maximum intensity (PMI). Although diastolic dysfunction may be present, it may not be detectable by resting physical examination. The constellation of a mildly displaced but sustained PMI and apical fourth heart sound, especially in the setting of hypertension, predisposes to, if not establishes, the presence of diastolic dysfunction.

Differential Diagnosis

The presence of dyspnea may represent cardiac, pulmonary, or comorbid disease. The differentiation often presents a challenge to the clinician, especially if there is a paucity of findings to support either a cardiac or pulmonary origin of dypnea. Familiarity of the potential cardiac causes that predispose to PVH will be helpful in deducing a cause of cardiac dyspnea or cardiac asthma.

Table 2 lists the cardiac conditions that predispose to heart failure. The table illustrates that many of the common causes of heart failure can lead to either heart failure with reduced ejection fraction or preserved ejection fraction.

IMAGING AND LABORATORY DATA

In decompensated or late stage heart disease, the history and physical examination may be adequate to establish the diagnosis of congestive heart failure; the diagnosis can be confirmed by laboratory data that will add prognostic data. However, in the early stages of heart disease, history and physical examination may be unremarkable, and laboratory assessment may be key in establishing the diagnosis.

Electrocardiogram

Despite its simplicity, the ECG remains an essential tool in the diagnosis of heart disease. The presence of increased voltage, especially with ST-T wave repolarization changes and findings of left atrial enlargement, is characteristic of left ventricular hypertrophy. Q waves may indicate a prior myocardial infarction and ischemic heart disease. Poor R wave progression (anterior QRS loop), nonspecific ST-T wave

Table 2
Common causes of heart failure

HFrEF (Systolic)	HFpEF (Diastolic)
Coronary artery disease	Coronary artery disease
Hypertension	Hypertension
Valvular heart disease	Valvular heart disease
Obstructive	Obstructive
Regurgitant	Regurgitant
Familial/genetic disorders	Amyloidosis
Hemochromatosis	Hemochromatosis
Toxic or drug-induced	
Anthracyclines	
Alcohol	
Cocaine	
Idiopathic dilated cardiomyopathy	
Pregnancy	
Endocrine/metabolic	Endocrine
Thryroid	Thryroid
Pheochromocytoma	Pheochromocytoma
Viral or other infectious agents (human immunodeficiency virus)	
Sarcoidosis	Sarcoidosis
Tachyarrhythmia	
Muscular dystrophy	
Obesity	Obesity
Myocarditis	

changes, left atrial enlargement, and nonspecific intraventricular conduction defect may be seen in nonischemic cardiomyopathy. The presence of atrial fibrillation may indicate tachycardia-induced cardiomyopathy. Sinus tachycardia in the setting of heart disease may represent decompensated congestive heart failure and portends a poor prognosis. The presence of a left bundle branch block indicates structural heart disease and is a common finding in nonischemic cardiomyopathy.

Chest Radiograph

The chest radiograph is another universally available imaging modality in the diagnosis of heart disease. The findings on chest radiograph may range from a pattern of chronic heart failure (enlarged heart, Kerley B lines, pleural effusions, and cephalization of pulmonary veins) to the pulmonary edema of acute heart failure. Different cardiac silhouettes may distinguish different causes of heart disease, such as left ventricular hypertrophy or rheumatic heart disease. The presence of a normal cardiac silhouette and cephalization of pulmonary veins that indicates PVH should raise the suspicion of diastolic dysfunction.

Echocardiogram

Doppler and 2-dimensional echocardiography is probably the most informative and cost-effective tool for the diagnosis of heart disease. Echocardiography can diagnose multiple heart conditions by establishing both global systolic and diastolic dysfunction, analyzing regional wall motion, evaluating valve function, estimating left ventricular filling pressures and pulmonary pressures, and assessing pericardial disease. In those patients who present a diagnostic dilemma, the echocardiogram assessment of chamber size and diastolic function may detect diastolic dysfunction.

Common Serum and Urine Laboratory Tests

Laboratory tests can help to establish the cause of heart disease, assist in management, establish prognosis, and identify reversible causes.

Useful diagnostic tests include ferritin, thyroid stimulating hormone, serum protein electrophoresis, urinalysis for catecholamines, and biomarkers of cardiac injury.

Basic and comprehensive metabolic panels offer useful information regarding electrolytes, renal function, and hepatic function. Hyponatremia (sodium <135 mEq/L) is a common finding in approximately 30% of heart failure patients.[18] A complete blood count may detect an elevated white count of infection or low hemoglobin level of anemia.

B-type naturetic peptide (BNP) is a counterregulatory hormone that is secreted by the ventricles in response to increased volume or pressure. BNP offers a useful adjunct to clinical assessment of dyspnea. BNP has been shown to distinguish cardiac from pulmonary dyspnea.[19] A normal BNP (<100 pg/mL) has an excellent negative predictive value in excluding cardiac dyspnea, and a BNP greater than 400 pg/mL has a high positive predictive value in confirming dyspnea due to heart failure.[19]

Cardiopulmonary Exercise Test

The cardiopulmonary exercise test may represent the most complete study available to assess dyspnea whose origin is not clinically apparent. By coupling external (pulmonary) respiration to internal (cellular) respiration, the test is able to distinguish exertional intolerance and dyspnea from pulmonary, cardiac, gas exchange, and deconditioning etiologies. Unfortunately, the test is not readily available in the community.

Table 3
Heart failure therapies

Therapy	Symptom Reduction	Mortality Benefit	Prevents Progression	Reduces Hospitalization	Population Targeted
Diuretics	Yes	No	No	Yes	Pulmonary congestion
ACE inhibitors	Yes	Yes	Yes	Yes	All
ARBs	Yes	Yes	Yes	Yes	ACE intolerant
β-blockers	Yes	Yes	Yes	Yes	NYHA FC II–IV (? all)
Digoxin	Yes	No	No	Yes	AF or sx after triple Rx
Spironolactone	Yes	Yes	Yes	Yes	NYHA III–IV, EF <35%
Calcium channel blockers	Yes	No	No	No	HTN and angina
Nitrates + hydralazine	Yes	Yes	?	?	Intolerant of ACE/ARB
Anticoagulation	No	No	No	No	AF or LV thrombus
Antiarrhythmics	?	Trend (amiodarone)	No	?	EP selected patients
AICD	No	Yes	No	No	Post MI EF <35% Selected patients
Cardiac resynchronization	Yes	No	Yes	Yes	QRS >130 msec, EF <35%, NYHA III–IV

Abbreviations: AF, atrial fibrillation; AICD, automatic implantable cardioverter defibrillator; ARB, angiotensin receptor blocker; EF, ejection fraction; EP, electrophysiology; FC, functional class; HTN, hypertension; LV, left ventricular; MI, myocardial infarction; NYHA, New York Heart Association.

Data from Petty TL, Seebass JS, editors. Pulmonary disorders of the elderly: diagnosis, prevention, and treatment. Philadelphia: ACP; 2007.

Cardiac Computed Tomography and Magnetic Resonance Imaging

The cardiac computed tomography may be a useful noninvasive assessment of cardiac anatomy and circulation in the evaluation of cardiomyopathy of unknown cause, especially to exclude ischemic heart disease. Cardiac magnetic resonance scan is able to assess anatomy, valve function, pericardial disease, and cardiomyopathy, including sarcoidosis. These tests are used only in selected patients.

Right and Left Heart Catheterization

Cardiac catheterization may be useful in selected patients to establish the diagnosis and extent of structural heart disease, (including ischemic and valvular heart disease) assessment of hemodynamics, and to direct and optimize therapy.

THERAPY

A detailed discussion of heart failure management is beyond the scope of this article. The reader is referred to one of the many excellent heart failure textbooks on the subject.

The management of heart failure is directed at the relief or amelioration of symptoms, the improvement of left ventricular function, and the prolongation of life. Therapy options have advanced significantly because the neurohormonal model has become widely accepted.[20] Effective therapies now include nonpharmacologic therapies such as exercise and cardiac rehabilitation; pharmaceutical therapies such as ACE inhibitors and β-blockers; and mechanical therapies such as implantable defibrillators, biventricular pacing, left ventricular assist devices, and cardiac transplantation. **Table 3** details some of the available therapeutic modalities, benefit, and patient populations targeted.

SUMMARY

Cardiac dyspnea, especially if present only with exercise, is often confused with asthma and exercise-induced bronchospasm. Cardiac dyspnea or asthma is the consequence of pulmonary edema due to PVH and not due to asthmatic bronchoconstriction. In overt, acute congestive heart failure, the diagnosis may be readily made by history and physical examination and pertinent laboratory and imaging data. However, in the early stages of heart disease, especially diastolic dysfunction, the diagnosis of cardiac dyspnea may be more elusive. The practicing physician must cull the history and physical examination for clues and order appropriate laboratory and imaging studies to establish the diagnosis of cardiac dyspnea. In distinguishing cardiac from pulmonary dyspnea, the most useful and informative studies include a serum BNP, echocardiogram, and if necessary, cardiopulmonary stress test.

REFERENCES

1. Lombardo TA, Harrison TR. Cardiac asthma. Circulation 1951;4:920.
2. Osler W. Angina pectoris and allied states. New York: D. Appleton; 1901.
3. Gehlbach BK, Geppert E. The pulmonary manifestations of left heart failure. Chest 2004;125(2):669.
4. West JB, Dollery CT, Naimark A. Distribution of blood flow in isolated lung: relation to vascular and alveolar pressures. J. Appl Physiol 1969;26:65.
5. Glazier JB, Hughes JMB, Maloney JE, et al. Measurements of capillary dimensions and blood volume in rapidly frozen lungs. J. Appl Physiol 1969;26:65.

6. Matthay MA, Martin TR. Pulmonary edema and acute lung injury. In: Murray JF, Nadel JA, Mason RJ, et al, editors. Textbook of respiratory medicine. 5th edition. Philadelphia: WB Saunders Company; 2010. p. 1283–355.

7. Jacobson JR, Garcia JG. Pulmonary circulation and regulation of fluid balance. In: Murray JF, Nadel JA, Mason RJ, et al, editors. Textbook of respiratory medicine. 5th edition. Philadelphia: WB Saunders Company; 2010. p. 108–33.

8. Uhley HN, Leeds SE, Sampson JJ, et al. Role of pulmonary lymphatics in chronic pulmonary edema. Circ Res 1962;11:966.

9. Costello ML, Mathieu-Costello O, West JB. Stress failure of alveolar epithelial cells studied by scanning electron microscopy. Am Rev Respir Dis 1992;145:1446.

10. Ware LB, Matthay MA. Clinical practice. Acute pulmonary edema. N Engl J Med 2005;353:2788.

11. Dimopoulou I, Daganou M, Tsintzas OK, et al. Effects of severity of long-standing congestive heart failure on pulmonary function. Respir Med 1998;92:1321.

12. Wood TE, McLeod P, Anthonisen NR, et al. Mechanics of breathing in mitral stenosis. Am Rev Respir Dis 1971;104:52.

13. Snashall PD, Chung KF. Airway obstruction and bronchial hyperresponsiveness in left ventricular failure and mitral stenosis. Am Rev Respir Dis 1991;144:945.

14. Mustafa KY, Nour MM, Shuhaiber H, et al. Pulmonary function before and sequentially after valve replacement surgery with correlation to preoperative hemodynamic data. Am Rev Respir Dis 1984;130:400.

15. Ravenscraft SA, Gross CR, Kubo SH, et al. Pulmonary function after successful heart transplantation. Chest 1993;103:54.

16. Hawkins NM, Petrie MC, Pardeep SJ, et al. Heart failure and chronic pulmonary disease: diagnostic pitfalls and epidemiology. Eur J Heart Fail 2009;11:130.

17. Levy D, Larson MG, Vasan RS, et al. The progression from hypertension to congestive heart failure. JAMA 1996;275:1557.

18. ADHERE Scientific Advisory Committee. Acute Decompensated Heart Failure Registry (ADHERE) core module Q1 2006 final cumulative national benchmark report. Mountain View, CA: Scios, Inc; 2006.

19. Maisel AS, Krishnaswamy P, Nowak RM, et al. Rapid measurement of B-type natriuretic peptide in the emergency diagnosis of heart failure. N Engl J Med 2002;347:161.

20. Mann DL, Bristow MR. Mechanisms and models in heart failure: The biomechanical and beyond. Circulation 2005;111:2837.

Allergic Rhinitis and Chronic Rhinosinusitis

Their Impact on Lower Airways

Jeevan B. Ramakrishnan, MD[a], Todd T. Kingdom, MD[b],
Vijay R. Ramakrishnan, MD[b],*

KEYWORDS

- Unified airway • Inflammation • Sinusitis • Asthma • Nasal polyps

KEY POINTS

- Several inflammatory mechanisms exist that connect the upper and lower airways through infectious, allergic, and nonallergic pathways.
- Patients with the most severe disease will benefit from thorough consideration, workup, and management of coexisting upper and lower airway disease.
- Long-lasting benefits may be achieved for lower airway disease with aggressive management of the upper airways.
- Surgical treatment of the nose and sinuses is known to improve nasal airflow, sleep quality, sense of smell, and sinonasal symptoms. There are also anatomic benefits that facilitate topical drug distribution, and the potential for decreased systemic inflammation related to the underlying disease.

INTRODUCTION

The notion that coincident inflammation commonly affects both the upper and lower airways via similar mechanisms has been well established. This idea has been reinforced over recent years with both basic and clinical research findings as well as with clinical observation.

Chronic airway inflammation commonly presents clinically as allergic rhinitis (AR) and chronic rhinosinusitis (CRS) in the upper airway, and as asthma in the lower airway. These conditions often coexist in the same patient, and are seen by a variety of general and specialty practitioners including family physicians, pediatricians, internists, pulmonologists, allergists, and otolaryngologists, as well as mid-level providers

Disclosures: V.R.R. is a Research Consultant (Arthrocare).
[a] Capitol Ear, Nose, and Throat, PA, Raleigh, NC, USA; [b] Department of Otolaryngology, University of Colorado, 12631 East 17th Avenue, B205, Aurora, CO 80045, USA
* Corresponding author. Department of Otolaryngology, University of Colorado, 12631 East 17th Avenue, B205, Aurora, CO 80045.
E-mail address: vijay.ramakrishnan@ucdenver.edu

Immunol Allergy Clin N Am 33 (2013) 45–60
http://dx.doi.org/10.1016/j.iac.2012.10.009
0889-8561/13/$ – see front matter © 2013 Elsevier Inc. All rights reserved.

immunology.theclinics.com

such as nurses and physician assistants. The incidence and prevalence of these disorders are high, and for allergy and asthma appear to be increasing over time. In addition, it is common for patients complaining of upper airway symptoms to have their lower airway overlooked, and vice versa.

Because of these factors, it is important for clinicians to be aware of the relationship between these disorders and how they can affect one another, to ensure optimal diagnosis and treatment. In patients with asthma, it is important to also evaluate the upper airway for symptoms and signs of AR and/or CRS. Diagnosing and treating these upper airway disorders can have a direct impact on lower airway inflammation and are important for optimizing patient outcomes. The impact on the lower airway of these upper airway conditions and their treatment are discussed here in detail.

UNIFIED AIRWAY THEORY

The unified airway theory has several suppositions.[1] First, pathophysiologic mechanisms ought to be similar despite the distance between the upper and lower airways. Anatomically the upper and lower airways are lined entirely with the same respiratory type of ciliated, pseudostratified columnar epithelium, which includes the mucosa of the middle ear, nose, sinuses, larynx, trachea, and down to the distal bronchioles. The unified airway theory considers these distinct anatomic units as a single functional unit. Continuing along this line of reason, when a pathophysiologic process, such as inflammation, affects one anatomic unit, the same process can be stimulated in another anatomic unit. This phenomenon can occur because of a local or systemic stimulus, and presents clinically when a patient with AR and asthma presents with worsening wheezing and chest tightness after an allergy exacerbation with increased nasal obstruction. The second postulate of the unified airway theory is that as the severity of airway disease fluctuates, both the upper and lower airways are affected to similar degrees. This notion implies that when effective treatment is initiated for upper airway symptoms, lower airway symptoms are expected to improve, and vice versa. Basic science and translational clinical research have largely supported these theories.[1] Understanding the pathophysiologic mechanisms affecting the respiratory system is essential for better understanding of how to optimally treat these patients. It is beyond the scope of this article to thoroughly review the concepts of the unified airway theory, but the general concept is presented as an underlying framework for the remainder of the article.

RHINITIS AND LOWER AIRWAYS

The understanding of the relationship between rhinitis and asthma has evolved over the years to reveal some important associations. Many studies have shown that patients with rhinitis often have coexisting asthma, and that treatment of rhinitis can improve the control of asthma. In this section, the epidemiology, pathophysiology, and clinical relevance are explored in detail.

Epidemiology

AR occurs with a prevalence of somewhere between 15% and 40%,[2] making it one of the most prevalent conditions among the general population. Asthma is estimated to affect about 7% of the general population.[2] As many as 38% of patients with AR have been shown to have concurrent asthma.[3] Overall, the epidemiologic data suggest that these conditions occur together more frequently than expected for either condition alone. In addition, several studies have shown that patients diagnosed with rhinitis have a significantly increased risk of developing asthma over time.[4–6]

In patients diagnosed with asthma, concurrent rhinitis is likewise a very common finding, occurring somewhere between 50% and 85% of the time. This finding is important, as patients with asthma and rhinitis appear to have more severe asthma in comparison with patients with asthma alone. Studies have shown increased cost of medical care and increased need for hospitalization in such patients with concomitant rhinitis and asthma.[7–10] These findings highlight the importance of evaluating the upper airway in patients with asthma.

Pathophysiology

As already mentioned, the histology of the upper airway from the nose to the bronchioles is identical. It follows logically that inflammation would affect these anatomically distinct areas in a similar fashion, at least at a cellular level. It has indeed been shown that the inflammatory cascade of lymphocytes, eosinophils, cytokines, and other inflammatory mediators share a similar profile, whether they occur in the upper or lower airway.[11–13] In addition, inflammation in the upper and lower airways is often caused by the same airborne irritants, such as pollutants or allergens, suggesting similar pathophysiologic mechanisms. Indeed, it has been demonstrated that patients with rhinitis have increased bronchial reactivity, even without a diagnosis of asthma.[14,15] Additional studies have looked at inflammatory markers in the upper and lower airways.[16–18] When allergic patients are stimulated with nasal provocation, changes include eosinophilia in the bronchial mucosa, elevated cytokine levels, and decreased peak expiratory flow when compared with nonallergic controls. Conversely, bronchial provocation of allergic patients causes an increase in cytokines, such as interleukin (IL)-5, eotaxin, and eosinophils, in nasal mucosa. These studies demonstrate that rhinitis and asthma are linked in their pathophysiology and can be thought of as different manifestations of a similar reactive airway disease.

Treatment

If inflammation of the upper airway can stimulate the same process in the lower airway, and vice versa, it seems possible that treatment of such inflammation could work the same way. However, the results of studies investigating this concept are mixed. Nevertheless, several studies have shown that treatment of patients with asthma with intranasal steroid spray for rhinitis resulted in fewer visits to the emergency department, fewer lost work days, and improved sleep quality.[19–22] There is also convincing evidence that treatment of rhinitis in children with immunotherapy reduces bronchial reactivity and the risk of subsequently developing asthma.[23]

Summary

Patients with rhinitis are at increased risk of developing asthma, and most patients with asthma have rhinitis. The pathophysiology of these conditions is closely related, and may in fact be different manifestations of the same disease process. Health care providers must be aware of this relationship, and must evaluate for both of these conditions when evaluating a patient for upper or lower airway complaints, as early recognition and appropriate treatment can improve quality of life, save costs, and prevent future morbidity.

CHRONIC RHINOSINUSITIS AND LOWER AIRWAYS

CRS can potentially contribute to lower airway disease through infectious mechanisms, such as in chronic bronchitis, bronchiectasis, or mucociliary dysfunction. In addition, inflammatory or neurogenic pathways may link CRS to lower airway disease in asthma, aspirin-exacerbated respiratory disease (AERD), and chronic cough. In certain cases, therapy for CRS can be expected to yield measurable benefits for the lower airways.

Epidemiology

CRS is responsible for nearly 20 million physician office visits per year.[24] This condition is increasing in prevalence and incidence with time, and its detrimental effects on quality of life and daily functioning are well accepted. Quality-of-life impairments in CRS patients are comparable in severity with those in disease states such as congestive heart failure, chronic obstructive pulmonary disease, and chronic low back pain.[25] Approximately $200 million per year are being spent on prescription medication, and $2 billion per year on nonprescription medication, to treat symptoms of sinusitis. There are also indirect accumulated costs, including time away from work/school and the associated loss of productivity. In the United States overall, CRS results in almost $4 billion of direct health care costs per year, and almost $6 billion of direct and indirect costs per year.[26,27]

Pathophysiology

CRS is no longer considered purely an infectious disease, but can be thought of as a multifactorial disease process of continued inflammation whereby infection may play a role in the initiation or sustenance of inflammation (**Tables 1** and **2**).[28]

Diagnosis of CRS

Over the past 20 years there has been a steady increase in clinical interest and research on rhinosinusitis. More recently, the quality of this research has steadily improved to include higher levels of evidence and more sophisticated methods of study. Beginning in 1996, there has been an evolving effort by the American Academy of Otolaryngology—Head and Neck Surgery, the American Rhinologic Society, the American Academy of Otolaryngic Allergy, and other collaborating, multidisciplinary organizations to define the diagnostic criteria for sinusitis. The modern definition was put forth in 2004 by a multidisciplinary task force, describing CRS in adults as "a group of disorders characterized by inflammation of the mucosa of the nose and paranasal sinuses of at least 12 weeks' duration."[26] The diagnosis is made by eliciting a combination of symptoms from the patient, as well as some form of confirmatory physical findings, as it is well known that diagnosis of CRS based on symptoms alone has a high false-positive rate (**Table 3**).

In addition to characteristic symptoms, objective evidence of disease is required to establish the diagnosis. Potential findings on nasal endoscopy may include discolored drainage, nasal polyps, and mucosal edema or erythema in the middle meatus. Alternatively, if no abnormalities are found on examination, noncontrast computed tomography (CT) can be used to confirm the diagnosis if bony and/or mucosal changes are demonstrated. This method of diagnosis by using a combination of subjective and objective findings has increased in accuracy since its introduction, and is the current recommended method.[28,29]

A few lessons on initial CRS diagnosis that can be gleaned from recent work are worthy of mention. Ideally an accurate history and physical examination would reliably predict the presence of CRS without the need for CT scan; however, AR and headache disorders can mimic many of the symptoms used for diagnosis. Amine and colleagues[30] have demonstrated that the more symptoms present, the more reliable the diagnosis, suggesting that in patients with many symptoms, objective confirmation with endoscopy or CT scan may not be absolutely required. Conversely, in patients

Table 1
Diagnostic subgroups of distinct types of rhinosinusitis and implicated inflammatory mediators

Classification	Subtypes	Inflammatory Categorization	Selected Inflammatory Mediators
Acute rhinosinusitis	Viral	T_H1, neutrophilic	IL-1β, -6, -8
	Nonviral		TNF-α
CRS without NP	Anatomic obstruction	T_H1, neutrophilic	IL-1β, -6, -8
	Bacterial		IFN-γ, TNF-α, TGF-β, GM-CSF, ICAM-1, MPO, MMR, TLR,
	Inflammatory without eosinophilia		MUC 5AC/B/8
CRS with NP	AFS	T_H2, eosinophilic	IL-5, -13
	AFS-like (without fungus)		IgE, TGF-β, MMP 7/9, MUC 1/4/8, VCAM-1, VEGF, GM-CSF,
	Eosinophilic CRS		eotaxin, RANTES, periostin, osteopontin, leukotrienes
	Gram-negative sinusitis with NP		
	Aspirin-exacerbated respiratory disease		

Abbreviations: AFS, allergic fungal sinusitis; CRS, chronic rhinosinusitis; GM-CSF, granulocyte macrophage colony-stimulating factor; ICAM, intercellular adhesion molecule; IFN, interferon; IgE, immunoglobulin E; IL, interleukin; MMP, matrix metalloproteinase; MMR, macrophage mannose receptor; MPO, myeloperoxidase; MUC, mucin; NP, nasal polyps; RANTES, regulated and normal T-cell expressed and secreted; TGF, transforming growth factor; TLR, toll-like receptor; TNF, tumor necrosis factor; VCAM, vascular cell adhesion molecule; VEGF, vascular endothelial growth factor.

Adapted from Timperley D, Schlosser RJ, Harvey RJ. Chronic rhinosinusitis: an education and treatment model. Otolaryngol Head Neck Surg 2010;143 (5 Suppl 3):S3–8.

Table 2
Etiologic factors in CRS

Environmental Factors	Local Host Factors	Systemic Host Factors
Smoking	Anatomic abnormality	Atopy
Pollution	Persistent local inflammation	Mucosal hyperreactivity
Allergens	Biofilms	Immune deficiency
Nonspecific particulate matter	Osteitis	Ciliary dysfunction
Microbes	Obstructing lesion	Cystic fibrosis
	Mucus character, innate immune function	Stress

Adapted from Kennedy DW, Ramakrishnan VR. Functional endoscopic sinus surgery: concepts, surgical indications, and techniques. In: Kennedy DW, Hwang PH, editors. Rhinology: diseases of the nose, sinuses and skull base. Thieme; 2012;306.

who have relatively few CRS symptoms and negative endoscopy, or in those whose primary complaint is headache, point-of-care CT scan frequently rules out CRS and eliminates the need for unnecessary empiric medical therapies, which are destined for failure and have associated costs and side effects.[31,32]

CRS Subtypes

As a multifactorial, chronic, inflammatory condition, significant heterogeneity may exist within this diagnostic group. In general, CRS can be divided into disease without nasal polyps (CRSsNP) and with nasal polyps (CRSwNP) (see **Table 1**). Each of these groups can be subdivided into more specific groups depending on comorbid factors, such as the presence of allergy and/or asthma (or eosinophilic inflammatory features), presence of inflammatory reaction to fungal antigens, or presence of aspirin intolerance (AERD). These subtypes of CRS continue to evolve as our understanding of the pathophysiology expands, and they are important because they have the potential to direct specific treatment, provide prognostic information, and improve research study design. Using a clinical phenotype to classify CRS patients is clearly oversimplified and not optimal. The move toward defining the disease and categorizing patients based on molecular profile has begun and provides great hope for the development of improved treatment paradigms in the future.

Understanding these subtypes of CRS is also important when trying to understand the relationship between CRS and the lower airways. Of the various subtypes, it is CRSwNP (also known as chronic hyperplastic sinusitis with nasal polyps, or eosinophilic CRS) that is most closely related to lower airway disease. In CRSwNP there is

Table 3
Diagnostic criteria for CRS

Major Symptoms	Minor Symptoms	Objective Evidence
Nasal congestion	Halitosis	Nasal endoscopy
Nasal obstruction	Fatigue	CT scan
Facial pain/pressure/fullness	Dental pain	
Purulent discharge	Cough	
Hyposmia/anosmia	Ear pressure	

The diagnosis is probable with two or more major symptoms, or one major and two or more minor symptoms.

often, but not always, tissue eosinophilia and frequently peripheral eosinophilia. Nearly half of these patients also have inhalant allergies, about half have asthma, and up to one-third may exhibit aspirin intolerance.[26,28] Similar to the relationship between rhinitis and asthma, asthma and CRS coexist at a higher frequency than one would expect based on the prevalence of each condition alone (about 20% of patients with CRS have asthma, compared with 5–8% of the general population). In addition, patients with severe asthma are much more likely to have concomitant CRS.

AERD (Samter's triad) is a chronic inflammatory condition that consists of CRSwNP, asthma, and aspirin insensitivity, and serves as a dramatic model of how the upper and lower airways are related. These patients typically present in adulthood with progressive sinonasal symptoms and rapidly develop aspirin insensitivity and asthma that is severe in about 50% of cases. Histopathology of both the upper and lower airways in this disease shows mast cell activation, marked eosinophilia, epithelial disruption, and pro-inflammatory cytokine production.[33–36] Treatment of this condition is targeted at both upper and lower airway inflammation. Basic medical treatment includes standard asthma care, oral and intranasal steroids, antihistamines, and nasal saline irrigations. Aspirin desensitization and antileukotriene therapy has also been shown to provide additional clinical benefit in this scenario. Endoscopic sinus surgery is frequently required as an adjunct to control the CRS and nasal polyposis, which frequently recur despite aggressive treatment.

Histopathologic studies show striking similarities in the cellular processes between CRS and asthma, including eosinophilic infiltration, lymphocytic infiltration, major basic protein deposition, basement membrane thickening, goblet cell hyperplasia, mucus hypersecretion, subepithelial edema, epithelial damage, and submucosal gland formation. There are a variety of cytokines and inflammatory mediators common to both disease processes, including IL-4, IL-5, IL-13, eotaxin, intercellular adhesion molecule 1, and vascular cell adhesion molecule 1. This similarity is even more apparent when comparing nonallergic CRSwNP with nonallergic, or intrinsic, asthma.[33,35] Clinical studies have shown that among patients with asthma and CRS, the severity of the asthma tended to correlate with the severity of CRS based on CT-scan scores, lung function testing, eosinophil counts, and exhaled nitric oxide.[37,38]

Coinfection of Upper and Lower Airways

Patients frequently relate the history during an acute exacerbation that symptoms began with a sinus infection and quickly progressed to bronchitis. Such reporting has led to the supposition that the sinus infection and postnasal drip physically passes through the glottis and trachea into the lower airways. Although this direct infection mechanism is possible in the absence of cough reflex, it is unlikely that the infection truly drips from the sinuses into the lungs. However, nuclear medicine studies have shown trace amounts of silent aspiration of nasopharyngeal secretions that occurs in nearly half of normal and diseased patients.[39,40] Alternatively, lower airway symptoms may arise in a delayed fashion as a result of circulating systemic inflammatory mediators or from a common susceptibility to bacterial epithelial attachment and disease progression, given the histologic similarity of the upper and lower airway.

Bacterial and fungal cultures from the upper and lower airways have been most frequently studied in the cystic fibrosis population. Some studies have shown similar bacteria and even similar strains, whereas others have not found a correlation between the two sites.[41–44] In CRS populations without concomitant pulmonary disease, there is no correlation between sinus and pulmonary fungal culture.[45] It is likely that direct infection of the lower airways is not a true result of bacteria "dripping" from the sinuses, but that lower airway symptoms may result from coinfection or may be a reactive phenomenon to systemic or reflex neurogenic inflammation.

TREATMENT OF CRS

Further evidence for the linkage between CRS and asthma lies in the data showing the effect of treatment of CRS on asthma. Many studies have shown that medical and surgical treatment of CRS in patients with asthma results in improved asthma control in the form of improved symptom scores, improved pulmonary function tests, decreased use of asthma medications, and prolonged benefits lasting months to years[46–49] (also noted in the pediatric population).[50,51] However, the majority of these studies were not randomized or controlled.

Medical Management of CRS

Medical therapies are central to the management of CRS with and without nasal polyps. Although data are lacking for much of the pharmaceutical interventions, medical treatment of CRS often includes antibiotics, oral and intranasal steroids, nasal saline irrigations, and adjunctive treatments such as antihistamines and decongestants (**Table 4**). Newer targeted therapies, such as anti-IgE and anti-IL5 antibody therapy, is under study.

There is good evidence to support the use of topical corticosteroids in CRSwNP, particularly in the setting of eosinophilia. Regular use of intranasal steroids is known to decrease mucosal eosinophilia, reduce polyp size, and improve sinonasal symptoms.[52–54] The most commonly used medications for CRSsNP include oral steroids and oral antibiotics. However, recent evidence-based reviews have shown that there is poor evidence for these therapies as "shotgun" therapies for CRS, and treatments are better selected based on patient-specific disease characteristics.[55,56] Antileukotriene therapy is frequently used in patients with CRSwNP and lower airway disease, although well-designed studies are lacking. Improvements in smell, rhinorrhea, and nasal congestion were seen in patients with AERD receiving 16 weeks of zileuton when compared with controls.[57] Another study examined both zafirlukast (26 patients) and zileuton (10 patients) in the management of nasal polyposis,[58] reporting 72% subjective improvement and 50% objective improvement or stabilization of disease. Ragab and colleagues[59] looked at the use of montelukast as an add-on therapy to topical and inhaled corticosteroids in patients with asthma and nasal polyps, with and without AERD. These investigators found subjective and objective improvement

Table 4 Common medical therapies for CRS, and associated level of evidence		
Therapy	CRS Without NP	CRS with NP
Mucolytic	C	D
Saline rinse	C	D
Antibiotics	C	C
Topical steroid	A	A
Oral steroid	D	C
Decongestant	D	D
Immunotherapy	D	D
Proton-pump inhibitor	C	C

Data from Fokkens W, Lund V, Bachert C, et al. EAACI position paper on rhinosinusitis and nasal polyps executive summary. Allergy 2005;60:583–601.

in asthma and nasal polyps independent of AERD status. There appears to be a subgroup of patients with nasal polyps and asthma in whom leukotriene receptor antagonists are effective. Overall, antileukotriene medications seem to play a variable role in the management of select patients with nasal polyposis. For AERD patients, aspirin desensitization improves both short-term and long-term outcomes with regard to the sinuses and lower airway.[60–63] Many mechanisms for its actions are hypothesized and are currently under study.

Surgical Management of CRS and Nasal Polyps

In patients with continued symptoms despite appropriate use of medical therapies, consideration should be given to surgical intervention. Endoscopic sinus surgery (ESS) may consist of simple polypectomy or progressively more thorough techniques such as functional endoscopic sinus surgery (FESS) or, rarely, nasalization (**Table 5**). The FESS technique stresses mucosal preservation and complete dissection of the involved sinuses, including removal of bony partitions and inflammatory foci, as well as identification and possible enlargement of sinus ostia.[64] FESS is the most widely used approach for general CRS and CRSwNP, and most current studies are performed using this technique. Although rare, potential complications must be considered and include epistaxis, orbital injury, and skull-base penetration.[65] Surgical goals include the removal of diseased tissue from the ethmoid cells, improving sinus ventilation, preserving or improving mucociliary clearance, and improving postoperative topical drug distribution within the sinuses.[66–68]

Several surgical indications exist, and as has been learned, there are a wide variety of patients who fall under the diagnosis of CRS. In general, even when considering the range of patient subgroups, overall success rates for ESS have been reported to range from 85% to 97%.[66,69,70] It has been suggested in the past that the presence of nasal polyps is predictive of worse surgical outcome and poor response to therapy. However, recent prospective data have demonstrated the benefits of ESS in patients with and without nasal polyps.[59,71] Poetker and colleagues[72] reported on the subjective and objective outcomes of 43 polyp and 76 nonpolyp patients undergoing ESS. In this study all patients, regardless of polyp status, had significant improvement in both subjective and objective parameters. Of note, patients with polyps showed a greater degree of improvement than patients without polyps, despite worse preoperative and postoperative CT and endoscopy scores.

Table 5 Endoscopic sinus surgery techniques	
Polypectomy	Removal of nasal polyps, no surgical dissection of sinus tissues
Functional endoscopic sinus surgery	Mucosal preservation, removal of diseased sinus tissue and bone, consider enlargement of sinus ostia
Nasalization (radical sphenoethmoidectomy)	Middle turbinectomy, total ethmoidectomy with mucosal stripping
Minimally invasive surgical technique	Enlarging transition spaces without manipulation of ostia, minimal tissue removal
Balloon sinus surgery	Balloon catheter dilates transition spaces and ostia, no tissue removal

Before sinus surgery, patients with asthma should be asked about symptoms such as cough, wheezing, shortness of breath, and chest tightness. Their medication regimen should be reviewed. Frequent use of a rescue inhaler or oral steroid dose packs may indicate that the asthma is not well controlled and warrants further discussion among the treatment team, including the asthma/pulmonary specialist, otolaryngologist, and anesthesiologist, before proceeding with surgery. Obviously it is ideal to have asthma optimally controlled before surgery to minimize the risk of an anesthetic pulmonary complication. Preoperative treatment with oral steroids is often used to mitigate some of these risks by decreasing airway hyperreactivity. Postoperatively these patients also require extra consideration, as the upper airway has just been manipulated with surgery and could potentially exacerbate lower airway inflammation. It is helpful to minimize nasal packing as much as possible to maximize nasal respiration and the associated humidification. Postoperative oral steroids are also helpful in controlling both upper and lower airway inflammation. Finally, consideration should be given to overnight observation in an inpatient setting if there is concern for lower airway obstruction perioperatively.

SPECIFIC OUTCOMES MEASUREMENTS FOR SURGERY IN CRS
Symptoms

Only recently have several validated, rhinology-specific, patient-based quality-of-life measurements come into common use. Coincidentally, improvements in surgical technique have been credited with enhanced outcomes. Many older studies are now considered outdated, as they used irregular and/or poorly supported methodologies for measurements of disease severity and outcomes after intervention, as well as less refined surgical techniques.[73] Many of these studies used inconsistent and subjective outcomes, such as time to recurrence of disease or time to revision surgery.

CRS patients refractory to medical therapies seek improvements in several symptoms, namely nasal congestion, fatigue, headache, decreased sense of smell, and nasal drainage. In a prospective study of medical management for CRS, gains were demonstrated in all domains except headache.[74] In a separate study, visual analog symptom scores improved after surgery in all symptoms except headache, and had lasting improvements to the study end point of 18 months.[75] A multi-institutional prospective study was performed comparing the results of continued medical therapy versus surgery in CRS patients who failed initial medical management.[76] In this landmark study, a total of 115 patients were followed to the 12-month end point (50 patients in the medical management arm and 65 patients in the surgery arm). During the study period, 17 patients elected to cross over from the medical cohort to the surgical cohort, owing to continued symptom severity. All 3 cohorts showed symptom improvement at 12 months, but interestingly greater improvements were noted in the surgery and cross-over groups. This study not only found significantly better symptom control but also documented less medication usage and fewer missed work/school days in the group who underwent surgery.

Sense of smell has not been extensively studied in all patient groups. In a prospective study of CRS patients undergoing FESS, the Smell Identification Test was performed preoperatively, and at 6 and 12 months postoperatively.[77] The investigators found that patients with severe olfactory dysfunction had significant improvements with surgery, whereas those with milder dysfunction did not. Patients with nasal polyps, asthma, and/or aspirin sensitivity were more likely to be anosmic preoperatively. Of note, anosmic patients with nasal polyps had significant improvements in smell after surgery, whereas anosmic nonpolyp patients did not. In a recent study using the Sniffin' Sticks smell test on polyp patients who underwent FESS, the presence of AERD was found to significantly limit olfactory restoration in comparison with aspirin-tolerant patients.[78] At this point, it is difficult to predict the restoration of sense of smell with sinus surgery, but this is certainly an area of interest and ongoing research.

Objective Outcomes

It is important to examine objective measurements of disease in addition to subjective quality-of-life measurements, as the two may not always correlate. Objective measurements of disease include CT staging systems and nasal endoscopy scoring systems. When comparing CRSwNP and CRSsNP populations, polyp patients, not surprisingly, have worse disease preoperatively on both CT and nasal endoscopy scoring.[72] Both populations made significant improvements in CT and endoscopy after surgery; polyp patients improved more in the endoscopic score, but still remained worse than those without polyps owing to their worse starting point. When specifically comparing AERD polyp patients to aspirin-tolerant polyp patients, AERD patients generally had significantly worse preoperative CT and nasal endoscopy scores.[79] However, after ESS there was no difference between the two groups in their degree of improvement on nasal endoscopy at a mean follow-up of 18 months, suggesting that significant benefits can be obtained in AERD patients with surgery.

Effects on Asthma

Several studies have demonstrated the benefits of ESS on lower airway disease in patients with CRS and asthma.[80–82] The mechanism of this improvement is incompletely defined, but may be related to decreased systemic proinflammatory mediators, such as leukotriene E4.[83] Several retrospective analyses of polyp patients undergoing ESS have compared aspirin-sensitive with aspirin-tolerant patients, and have found ESS to improve sinus and asthma symptoms, improve nasal endoscopy scores, improve FEV1, and decrease the use of inhaled corticosteroids in both groups.[71,84,85] This issue has been of particular interest in patients with AERD, especially in terms of the durability of benefit. Long-term asthma outcomes were assessed by surveying 65 patients with AERD who underwent ESS, with a mean 10-year follow-up.[86] Out of 34 respondents, 29 (94%) patients with asthma preoperatively noticed a subjective asthma improvement at least 1 year postoperatively. Improvements were also noted in the use of oral and inhaled steroids, frequency of asthma attacks, frequency of physician visits for asthma-related concerns, and hospitalizations for asthma exacerbations.

SUMMARY

A clear link exists between the upper and lower airways, based on anatomy, pathophysiology, epidemiology, and disease severity. Medical therapies directed at the management of AR and CRS can be effective for both upper and lower airway symptoms. In addition, overall quality of life can be improved by concomitant management of both sites of disease. There is now strong evidence to support the value of surgery in CRS patients for sinonasal symptoms, but there are also several lower-level studies suggesting that ESS may benefit lower airway disease in a subset of patients. This finding does not imply that medical therapies should not be entertained, but rather that surgery can be considered an adjunct to medical therapies in refractory patients and that well-designed larger-scale studies should be performed in this patient population.

REFERENCES

1. Krouse J, Brown R, Fineman S, et al. Asthma and the unified airway. Otolaryngol Head Neck Surg 2007;136(Suppl 5):S75–106.
2. Meltzer EO. The relationships of rhinitis and asthma. Allergy Asthma Proc 2005; 26:336–40.
3. Corren J. Allergic rhinitis and asthma: how important is the link? J Allergy Clin Immunol 1997;99:S781–6.
4. Guerra S, Sherrill DL, Martinez FD, et al. Rhinitis as an independent risk factor for adult-onset asthma. J Allergy Clin Immunol 2002;109:419–25.
5. Greisner WA, Settipane RJ, Settipane GA. Co-existence of asthma and allergic rhinitis: a 23-year follow-up study of college students. Allergy Asthma Proc 1998;19:185–8.
6. Huovinen E, Kaprio J, Laitinen LA, et al. Incidence and prevalence of asthma among adult Finnish men and women of the Finnish twin cohort from 1975 to 1990, and their relation to hay fever and chronic bronchitis. Chest 1999;115: 928–36.
7. Yawn BP, Yunginger JW, Wollan PC, et al. Allergic rhinitis in Rochester, Minnesota residents with asthma: frequency and impact on health care charges. J Allergy Clin Immunol 1999;103:54–9.
8. Thomas M, Kocevar VS, Zhang Q, et al. Asthma-related health care resource use among asthmatic children with and without concomitant allergic rhinitis. Pediatrics 2005;115:129–34.
9. Kocevar VS, Bisgaard H, Jonsson L, et al. Variations in pediatric asthma hospitalization rates and costs between and within Nordic countries. Chest 2004;125: 1680–4.
10. Halpern MT, Schmier JK, Richner R, et al. Allergic rhinitis: a potential cause of increased asthma medication use, costs, and morbidity. J Asthma 2004;41(1): 117–26.
11. American Thoracic Society Workshop. Immunobiology of asthma and rhinitis: pathogenic factors and therapeutic options. Am J Respir Crit Care Med 1999; 160:1778–87.
12. Meltzer EO. Role for cysteinyl leukotrienes receptor antagonist therapy in asthma and their potential role in allergic rhinitis based on the concept of "one airway linked disease." Ann Allergy Asthma Immunol 2000;84:176–87.
13. Pawankar R. Allergic rhinitis and asthma: are they manifestations of one syndrome? Clin Exp Allergy 2006;36:1–4.
14. Prieto J, Gutierrez V, Berto JM, et al. Sensitivity and maximal response to methacholine in perennial and seasonal allergic rhinitis. Clin Exp Allergy 1996;26: 61–7.
15. European Community Respiratory Health Survey II Steering Committee. The European Community Respiratory Health Survey II. Eur Respir J 2002;20:1071–9.
16. Braunstahl GJ, Kleinjan A, Overbeek SE, et al. Segmental bronchial provocation induces nasal inflammation in allergic rhinitis patients. Am J Respir Crit Care Med 2000;161:2051–7.
17. Braunstahl GJ, Overbeek SE, Kleinjan A, et al. Nasal allergen provocation induces adhesion molecule expression and tissue eosinophilia in upper and lower airways. J Allergy Clin Immunol 2001;107:469–76.
18. Braunstahl GJ, Overbeek SE, Fokkens WJ, et al. Segmental bronchoprovocation in allergic rhinitis patients affects mast cell and basophil numbers in nasal and bronchial mucosa. Am J Respir Crit Care Med 2001;164:858–65.

19. Stelmach R, do Patrocinio T, Nunes M, et al. Effect of treating allergic rhinitis with corticosteroids in patients with mild-to moderate persistent asthma. Chest 2005; 128:3140–7.
20. Watson WT, Becker AB, Simons FE. Treatment of allergic rhinitis with intranasal corticosteroids in patients with mild asthma: effect on lower airway responsiveness. J Allergy Clin Immunol 1993;91:97–101.
21. Taramarcaz P, Gibson PG. Intranasal corticosteroids for asthma control in people with coexisting asthma and rhinitis. Cochrane Database Syst Rev 2003;(3): CD003570. http://dx.doi.org/10.1002/14651858.CD003570.
22. Thio BJ, Slingerland GL, Fredriks AM, et al. Influence of intranasal steroids during the grass pollen season on bronchial responsiveness in children and young adults with asthma and hay fever. Thorax 2000;55:826–32.
23. Möller C, Dreborg S, Ferdousi HA, et al. Pollen immunotherapy reduces the development of asthma in children with seasonal rhinoconjunctivitis (the PAT study). J Allergy Clin Immunol 2002;109:251–6.
24. Mattos JL, Woodard CR, Payne SC. Trends in common rhinologic illnesses: analysis of U.S. healthcare surveys 1995-2007. Int Forum Allergy Rhinol 2011;1(1):1–10.
25. Gliklick RE, Metson R. The health impact of chronic sinusitis seeking otolaryngologic care. Otolaryngol Head Neck Surg 1995;113:104–9.
26. Benninger MS, Ferguson BJ, Hadley JA, et al. Adult chronic rhinosinusitis: definitions, diagnosis, epidemiology and pathophysiology. Otolaryngol Head Neck Surg 2003;129(Suppl 3):S1–32.
27. Meltzer EO, Hamilos DL, Hadley JA, et al. Rhinosinusitis: establishing definitions for clinical research and patient care. Otolaryngol Head Neck Surg 2004;131: S1–62.
28. Fokkens W, Lund V, Mullol J, et al. European position paper on rhinosinusitis and nasal polyps (EPOS). Rhinol Suppl 2012;23(3):1–298.
29. Bhattacharyya N, Lee LN. Evaluating the diagnosis of chronic rhinosinusitis based on clinical guidelines and endoscopy. Otolaryngol Head Neck Surg 2010;143:147–51.
30. Amine M, Lininger L, Fargo KN, et al. Outcomes of endoscopy and computed tomography in patients with chronic rhinosinusitis. Int Forum Allergy Rhinol 2012. [Epub ahead of print].
31. Leung R, Kern R, Jordan N, et al. Upfront computed tomography scanning is more cost-beneficial than empiric medical therapy in the initial management of chronic rhinosinusitis. Int Forum Allergy Rhinol 2011;1(6):471–80.
32. Tan BK, Chandra RK, Conley DB, et al. A randomized trial examining the effect of pretreatment point-of-case computed tomography imaging on the management of patients with chronic rhinosinusitis symptoms. Int Forum Allergy Rhinol 2011; 1(3):229–34.
33. Dhong H, Hyo K, Cho D. Histopathologic characteristics of chronic sinusitis with bronchial asthma. Acta Otolaryngol 2005;125:169–76.
34. Harlin S, Ansel D, Lane S, et al. A clinical and pathologic study of chronic sinusitis: the role of the eosinophil. J Allergy Clin Immunol 1988;81:867–75.
35. Ponikau J, Sherris D, Kephart G, et al. Features of airway remodeling and eosinophilic inflammation in chronic rhinosinusitis: is the histopathology similar to asthma? J Allergy Clin Immunol 2003;112:877–82.
36. Barrios R, Kheradmand F, Batts L, et al. Asthma: pathology and pathophysiology. Arch Pathol Lab Med 2006;130:447–51.
37. Bresciani M, Paradis L, Des Roches A, et al. Rhinosinusitis in severe asthma. J Allergy Clin Immunol 2001;107:73–80.

38. ten Brinke A, Grootendorst D, Schmidt J. Chronic sinusitis in severe asthma is related to sputum eosinophilia. J Allergy Clin Immunol 2002;109:621–6.
39. Huxley EJ, Viroslav J, Gray WR, et al. Pharyngeal aspiration in normal adults and patients with depressed consciousness. Am J Med 1978;64:564–9.
40. Ozagar A, Dede F, Turoglu HT, et al. Aspiration of nasal secretions into the lungs in patients with acute sinonasal infections. Laryngoscope 2000;110(1):107–10.
41. Bonestroo HJ, de Winter-de Groot KM, van der Ent CK, et al. Upper and lower airway cultures in children with cystic fibrosis: do not neglect the upper airways. J Cyst Fibros 2010;9(2):130–4.
42. Roby BB, McNamara J, Finkelsteing M, et al. Sinus surgery in cystic fibrosis patients: comparison of sinus and lower airway cultures. Int J Pediatr Otorhinolaryngol 2008;72(9):1365–9.
43. Muhlebach MS, Miller MB, Moore C, et al. Are lower airway or throat cultures predictive of sinus bacteriology in cystic fibrosis? Pediatr Pulmonol 2006;41(5): 445–51.
44. Godoy JM, Godoy AN, Ribalta G, et al. Bacterial pattern in chronic sinusitis and cystic fibrosis. Otolaryngol Head Neck Surg 2011;145(4):673–6.
45. Ragab A, Clement P, Vincken W, et al. Fungal cultures of different parts of the upper and lower airways in chronic rhinosinusitis. Rhinology 2006;44(1): 19–25.
46. Batra P, Kern R, Tripathi A, et al. Outcome analysis of endoscopic sinus surgery in patients with nasal polyps and asthma. Laryngoscope 2003;113:1703–6.
47. Slavin R. Asthma and sinusitis. J Allergy Clin Immunol 1992;90(3 Pt 2):534–7.
48. Jankowski R, Moneret-Vautrin DA, Goets R, et al. Incidence of medico-surgical treatment for nasal polyps on the development of associated asthma. Rhinology 1992;30:249–58.
49. Alobid I, Benitez P, Bernal-Sprekelsen M, et al. The impact of asthma and aspirin sensitivity on quality of life of patients with nasal polyposis. Qual Life Res 2005;14: 789–93.
50. Rachelefsky G, Katz RM, Siegel SC. Chronic sinus disease with associated reactive airway disease in children. Pediatrics 1984;73:526–9.
51. Friedman R, Ackerman M, Wald E, et al. Asthma and bacterial sinusitis in children. J Allergy Clin Immunol 1984;74:185–94.
52. Mastalerz L, Milewski M, Duplaga M, et al. Intranasal fluticasone propionate for chronic eosinophilic rhinitis in patients with aspirin-induced asthma. Allergy 1997;52:895–900.
53. Ogata Y, Okinaka Y, Takahashi M. Detection of activated eosinophils in nasal polyps of an aspirin-induced asthma patient. Rhinology 1997;37:16–20.
54. Nores JM, Avan P, Bonfils P. Medical management of nasal polyposis: a study in a series of 152 consecutive patients. Rhinology 2003;41:97–102.
55. Soler ZM, Oyer SL, Kern RC, et al. Antimicrobials and chronic rhinosinusitis with or without polyposis in adults: an evidence-based review with recommendations. Int Forum Allergy Rhinol 2012. [Epub ahead of print].
56. Poetker DM, Jakubowski LA, Lal D, et al. Oral corticosteroids in the management of adult chronic rhinosinusitis with and without nasal polyps: an evidence-based review with recommendations. Int Forum Allergy Rhinol 2012. [Epub ahead of print].
57. Dahlen B, Nizankowska E, Szczeklik A, et al. Benefits from adding the 5-lipoxygenase inhibitor zileuton to conventional therapy in aspirin-intolerant asthmatics. Am J Respir Crit Care Med 1998;157(4 pt 1):1187–94.
58. Parnes S, Chuma A. Acute effects of antileukotrienes on sinonasal polyposis and sinusitis. Ear Nose Throat J 2000;79:18–20, 24–5.

59. Ragab SM, Lund VJ, Scadding G. Evaluation of the medical and surgical treatment of chronic rhinosinusitis: a prospective, randomized, controlled trial. Laryngoscope 2004;114:923–30.
60. Stevenson DD. Aspirin desensitization in patients with AERD. Clin Rev Allergy Immunol 2003;24:159–68.
61. Stevenson DD, Hankammer M, Mathison D, et al. Aspirin desensitization treatment of aspirin-sensitive patients with rhinosinusitis-asthma: long term outcomes. J Allergy Clin Immunol 1996;98:751–8.
62. Gosepath J, Schafer D, Mann WJ. Aspirin sensitivity: long term follow-up after up to 3 years of adaptive desensitization using a maintenance dose of 100 mg of aspirin a day. Laryngorhinootologie 2002;81:732–8.
63. Rozsasi A, Polzehl D, Deutschle T, et al. Long-term treatment with aspirin desensitization: a prospective clinical trial comparing 100 and 300 mg aspirin daily. Allergy 2008;63:1228–34.
64. Kennedy DW, Zinreich SJ, Rosenbaum AE, et al. Functional endoscopic sinus surgery. Theory and diagnostic evaluation. Arch Otolaryngol 1985;111:576–82.
65. Ramakrishnan VR, Kingdom TT, Nayak JV, et al. Nationwide incidence of major complications in endoscopic sinus surgery. Int Forum Allergy Rhinol 2012;2(1):34–9.
66. Senior B, Kennedy D, Tanabodee J, et al. Long term results of functional endoscopic sinus surgery. Laryngoscope 1998;108:151–7.
67. Harvey RJ, Goddard JC, Wise SK, et al. Effects of endoscopic sinus surgery and delivery device on cadaver sinus irrigation. Otolaryngol Head Neck Surg 2008;139(1):137.
68. Wormald PJ, Cain T, Oates L, et al. A comparative study of three methods of nasal irrigation. Laryngoscope 2004;114(2):2224–7.
69. Levine HL. Functional endoscopic sinus surgery: evaluation, surgery, and follow-up of 250 patients. Laryngoscope 1990;100:79–83.
70. Poetker DM, Smith TL. Adult chronic rhinosinusitis: surgical outcomes and the role of endoscopic sinus surgery. Curr Opin Otolaryngol Head Neck Surg 2007;15:6–9.
71. Smith TL, Mendolia-Loffredo S, Loehrl TA, et al. Predictive factors and outcomes in endoscopic sinus surgery for chronic rhinosinusitis. Laryngoscope 2005;115:2199–205.
72. Poetker DM, Mendolia-Loffredo S, Smith TL. Outcomes of endoscopic sinus surgery for chronic rhinosinusitis associated with sinonasal polyposis. Am J Rhinol 2007;21:84–8.
73. Smith TL. Outcomes research in rhinology: chronic rhinosinusitis. ORL J Otorhinolaryngol Relat Spec 2004;66(4):202–6.
74. Hessler JL, Piccirillo JF, Fang D, et al. Clinical outcomes of chronic rhinosinusitis in response to medical therapy: results of a prospective study. Am J Rhinol 2007;21(1):10–8.
75. Soler ZM, Mace J, Smith TL. Symptom-based presentation of chronic rhinosinusitis and symptom-specific outcomes after endoscopic sinus surgery. Am J Rhinol 2008;22(3):297–301.
76. Smith TL, Kern RC, Palmer JN, et al. Medical therapy versus surgery for chronic rhinosinusitis: a prospective multi-institutional study with 1-year follow-up. Int Forum Allergy Rhinol 2012. [Epub ahead of print].
77. Litvack JR, Mace J, Smith TL. Does olfactory function improve after endoscopic sinus surgery. Otolaryngol Head Neck Surg 2009;140(3):312–9.

78. Katotomichelakis M, Riga M, Davris S, et al. Allergic rhinitis and aspirin-exacerbated respiratory disease as predictors of the olfactory outcome after endoscopic sinus surgery. Am J Rhinol Allergy 2009;23(3):348–53.

79. Robinson JL, Griest S, James KE, et al. Impact of aspirin intolerance on outcomes of sinus surgery. Laryngoscope 2007;117(5):825–30.

80. Nishioka GJ, Cook PR, Davis WE, et al. Function endoscopic sinus surgery in patients with chronic sinusitis and asthma. Otolaryngol Head Neck Surg 1994; 110:494–500.

81. Dunlop G, Scadding GK, Lund VJ. The effect of endoscopic sinus surgery on asthma: management of patients with chronic rhinosinusitis, nasal polyposis and asthma. Am J Rhinol 1999;13:261–5.

82. Uri N, Cohen-Kerem R, Barzilai G, et al. Functional endoscopic sinus surgery in the treatment of massive polyposis in asthmatic patients. J Laryngol Otol 2002; 116:185–9.

83. Higashi N, Taniguchi M, Mita H, et al. Clinical features of asthmatic patients with increased urinary leukotriene E4 excretion (hyperleukotrienuria): involvement of chronic hyperplastic rhinosinusitis with nasal polyposis. J Allergy Clin Immunol 2004;113(2):277–83.

84. Awad OG, Lee JH, Fasano MB, et al. Sinonasal outcomes after endoscopic sinus surgery in asthmatic patients with nasal polyps: a difference between aspirin-tolerant and aspirin-induced asthma? Laryngoscope 2008;118:1282–6.

85. Awad OG, Fasano MB, Lee JH, et al. Asthma outcomes after endoscopic sinus surgery in aspirin-tolerant versus aspirin-induced asthmatic patients. Am J Rhinol 2008;22:197–203.

86. Loehrl TA, Ferre RM, Toohill RJ, et al. Long-term asthma outcomes after endoscopic sinus surgery in aspirin triad patients. Am J Otolaryngol 2006;27: 154–60.

The Overlap of Bronchiectasis and Immunodeficiency with Asthma

Tho Truong, MD

KEYWORDS

- Bronchiectasis • Asthma • Immunodeficiency • Atopy • B lymphocyte
- T lymphocyte

KEY POINTS

- Bronchiectasis should be considered as both a differential diagnosis for, as well as a co-morbidity in, patients with asthma, especially severe or long-standing asthma.
- Chronic airway inflammation is thought to be the primary cause of bronchiectasis, as seen in chronic or recurrent pulmonary infections and autoimmune conditions that involve the airways.
- Consequently, immunodeficiencies with associated increased susceptibility to respiratory tract infections or chronic inflammatory airways also increase the risk of developing bronchiectasis.
- Chronic bronchiectasis is associated with impaired mucociliary clearance and increased bronchial secretions, leading to airway obstruction and airflow limitation, which can lead to the exacerbation of underlying asthma or an increase in asthma symptoms.

INTRODUCTION

Bronchiectasis should be considered as both a differential diagnosis for, as well as a comorbidity in, patients with asthma, especially severe or long-standing asthma. Chronic airway inflammation is thought to be the primary cause of bronchiectasis, as demonstrated in chronic or recurrent pulmonary infections and autoimmune conditions that involve the airways. Consequently, immunodeficiencies with associated increased susceptibility to respiratory tract infections or chronic inflammatory airways also increase the risk of developing bronchiectasis. Chronic bronchiectasis is associated with impaired mucociliary clearance and increased bronchial secretions, leading to airway obstruction and airflow limitation, which can lead to the exacerbation of underlying asthma or an increase in asthma symptoms.

The Definition of Bronchiectasis

Chronic and abnormal dilation of the airways characterizes bronchiectasis. This persistent enlargement of the bronchi results in decreased clearance of respiratory secretions,

Allergy and Clinical Immunology, National Jewish Health, Denver, CO, USA
E-mail address: truongt@njhealth.org

http://dx.doi.org/10.1016/j.iac.2012.10.007
0889-8561/13/$ – see front matter © 2013 Elsevier Inc. All rights reserved.
immunology.theclinics.com

which then may lead to symptoms of airflow obstruction and increased mucus production and retention. Airflow limitation in bronchiectasis may be reversible as well as fixed. These postobstructive changes further increase the risk of respiratory infection and inflammatory damage in the airways, which in turn can worsen the bronchiectasis. These conditions also produce an airway environment that predisposes to persistent abnormal colonization of microflora, further driving the bronchiectasis. In addition to infection and autoimmune disease, significant chronic aspiration of oropharyngeal or gastric contents as well as chronic exposure to toxic inhalants may also contribute to or result in bronchiectasis.

The Diagnosis of Bronchiectasis

The current defining test for bronchiectasis is radiographic, using high-resolution computed tomography (HRCT) of the chest. The patient's clinical history is also taken into account. A luminal airway diameter that is more than 1.5 times the adjacent blood vessel supports the presence of cylindrical bronchiectasis; a normal luminal airway diameter is usually 1.0 to 1.5 times the size of an adjacent vessel. Other features are also considered besides airways dilation, such as a lack of tapering of the airways when dilation is present, bronchial wall thickening in the dilated airways, the presence of cysts adjacent to the luminal wall of the dilated bronchiole, and mucopurulent plugs. When there is involvement of the smaller airways, there can be irregular, more peripherally located linear branch markings (2–4 mm), a so-called tree-in-bud pattern. Bronchial wall thickening has been suggested as the best predictor of functional decline, and the presence of cysts off of the bronchial wall may signal more destructive bronchiectasis. Although also described with emphysema, blebs can also appear more distally but are generally thinner in wall thickness and are not accompanied by proximal airway changes as seen in emphysema. Evidence for chronic infection, such as consolidation, lymphadenopathy, and vascular disruption, may also be seen.[1]

Bronchiectasis and Asthma

There have been many studies that demonstrate considerable overlap between asthma and bronchiectasis. For instance, investigators[2–4] studied 245 patients characterized as having severe asthma. Of these patients, 24.8% had radiographic evidence of bronchiectasis on CT of the chest. In another study of 1680 patients with a diagnosis of asthma, about 3% had radiographic bronchiectasis. In contrast to age- and gender-matched patients with asthma without bronchiectasis who generally had only mild intermittent or mild persistent asthma (69.4%), most of those patients with asthma with bronchiectasis had severe persistent asthma (49.0%). Not surprisingly, these patients had a much higher rate of pulmonary complications and hospitalizations for respiratory failure.[5]

Bronchiectasis and Immunodeficiency States

Because the presence of bronchiectasis may significantly alter the prognosis of patients with asthma, it is important to optimize the management of its known causes and contributors. There is some evidence to suggest that the diagnosis and treatment of underlying immunodeficiency can prevent or slow the deterioration of pulmonary outcomes in patients with bronchiectasis and certain immunodeficiency states. A longitudinal study of children with primary immunodeficiency showed that children diagnosed with bronchiectasis at a median age of 3 years and subsequently diagnosed with and treated for primary humoral immunodeficiency did not have deterioration of pulmonary function at 9 years of age, based on pulmonary function studies and HRCT scores.[6] Another study on the efficacy of intravenous immunoglobulin treatment in children with common variable immunodeficiency (CVID) found that treatment with a sufficient replacement dose of intravenous gamma globulin (IVIG) significantly reduced the mean number of respiratory infections per patient per year, from 10.2 to 2.5. The annual number and length of hospital stays per patient also decreased significantly from 1.36 to 0.21 admissions and 16.35 to 6.33 days, respectively. Additionally, the mean annual number of antibiotics used per patient decreased significantly from 8.27 to 2.50. These investigators suggested that age at diagnosis, diagnostic delay, number of respiratory tract infections, and number of antibiotics were found to be significantly higher in patients with bronchiectasis. Thus, an evaluation for immunodeficiency states should be considered in all patients with bronchiectasis to optimize its management and minimize adverse sequelae.

Immunodeficiency, Atopy, and Asthma

In addition to sinopulmonary infections playing a role in poorly controlled asthma, patients with certain primary and secondary immunodeficiency diagnoses also have an increased risk for atopic disease. For instance, up to 50% of children with selective immunoglobulin A (IgA) deficiency have been observed to have allergic disease.[7] In a prospective study of children with selective IgA or IgG4 subclass deficiency, the occurrence of allergic disease and asthma increased with decreased levels of IgA and/or IgG4 in serum and salivary IgA. Another study showed that not only was the prevalence of atopy higher in a group of children with selective IgA deficiency compared with the control population, but also that the children with selective IgA deficiency had more frequent concomitant airways hyperresponsivity to the dust mite *Dermatophagoides pteronyssinus*.[8–10] It is thought that deficient mucosal immunity in IgA deficiency plays a role in the dysregulation of tolerance to allergens.

Perhaps counter to intuition, even patients with profound defects in antibody production, including IgE, have demonstrated a relatively high incidence of asthma and atopic disease. In 2008, Shabestari and Rezaei[11] reported a case in which a patient with Bruton agammaglobulinemia, with essentially absent serum concentrations of all immunoglobulin isotypes and virtually absent CD19+ lymphocytes, had a positive skin prick test to multiple airborne allergens. He also had bronchial hyperresponsivity by allergen challenge and spirometry. It is speculated that a bias toward T-helper cell type 2 (Th2)-mediated immune response accounts for this.

This Th2-bias has also been suggested in patients with CVID through the demonstration of increased interleukin 4 (IL-4) and IL-10 production. A high incidence of asthma, usually diagnosed after the initial presentation, was seen in 83% of pediatric patients with CVID.[12] Similarly, in another study, 9 out of 18 patients who had a diagnosis of CVID and a clinical history suggestive of allergic asthma tested positive to bronchoprovocation with histamine or specific allergen challenge; 6 of those patients had positive placebo-controlled bronchoprovocation to a specific allergen despite negative allergen-specific IgE and skin testing.[13,14]

Patients with secondary immunodeficiency, such as human immunodeficiency virus (HIV) infection, have also demonstrated clinical atopy, and in some studies, increased IgE-mediated atopy. Some data support that patients who are HIV positive present with a higher incidence of atopy in the earlier stages of HIV infection compared with the general population. Multivariate analysis of 74 hospitalized patients with HIV demonstrated that a personal history suggestive of allergic disease and serum IgE level >150 ku/L were predictors of atopy; gender, HIV risk group, CD4+ T cells, CD23 expression on B cells, and AIDS were not associated.[15] This study speculated that because allergic reactions could accelerate HIV infection by increasing the type 2 cytokines, identifying the atopic state in patients with HIV, especially those with IgE greater than 150 ku/L or a personal history that suggests allergy, was important to optimizing control of the HIV infection.

Immunodeficiency

Both primary and secondary immunodeficiencies should be considered in patients with bronchiectasis. Both primary and secondary immunodeficiency can increase the risk for sinopulmonary infections, leading to bronchiectasis. The evaluation for immunodeficiency is guided by the clinical presentation, such as patient age and gender, past medical history, present health, nutritional status, as well as history of infections (including severity, infectious organisms, and involved organ systems).

Secondary Immunodeficiency

Systemic illnesses, such as diabetes, hematologic malignancies, and chronic infections; immunosuppressive treatments, such as chemotherapy and radiation; and protein-losing syndromes may cause secondary immunodeficiency. Secondary immunodeficiency may also occur in critically ill and older hospitalized patients because prolonged serious illness and poor or diminished nutrition can lead to impaired immune responses. Frequently, secondary immunodeficiency can be corrected if the underlying problem resolves.

Protein loss
Serum protein loss through the kidneys, gastrointestinal (GI) tract, or skin, as with severe burns or dermatitis, can lead to immunodeficiency, particularly because of the loss of IgG and albumin. Enteropathy can also result in lymphopenia with the loss of both T and B lymphocytes. In intestinal lymphangiectasia, there is abnormal dilatation of intestinal mucosal lymphatic channels, which leads to the loss of immunoglobulins and lymphocytes into the gut lumen. The disorder may be congenital or result from processes that obstruct lymph drainage of the gut or cause an increased central venous pressure. These disorders can mimic B- and T-cell deficiencies, but treatment with a diet high in medium-chain triglycerides may decrease the loss of immunoglobulins and markedly improve lymphocyte counts.

Nutrition
Undernutrition also impairs immune responses. It should be considered as a cause for immunodeficiency states, particularly in elderly, chronically ill, institutionalized, or homebound patients. Calcium, vitamin E, and zinc play essential roles in immunity. The risk for calcium deficiency is increased in the elderly because of decreased calcium absorption from the GI tract as well as decreased ingestion of calcium from the diet. Institutionalized or homebound elderly patients are also more likely to have zinc deficiency than the general population.

Immune function and aging
Normal decreases in immune function have been described in healthy aging patient populations. For instance, cellular immunity may be reduced because the thymus generally produces fewer naïve T cells. The total number of T lymphocytes does not decrease, but naïve T cells potentiate the response to new antigens. The preexisting T-cell repertoire can only recognize a limited number of antigens. In addition, impaired cellular signal transduction has been demonstrated, and this could lead to decreased signaling to B cells to make antibodies and decrease the T-cell response to antigen.

Neutrophils are also less effective in phagocytosis and have decreased microbicidal activity.

Hematological malignancies

Although hematologic malignancy has been reported in up to 30% of patients with primary immunodeficiencies, secondary immunodeficiency can be seen in patients with primary lymphoproliferative disorders. Cellular and humoral immune deficiencies have been described in acute and chronic leukemias, myeloma, and lymphomas. Because these conditions can result in B and T lymphocyte dysfunction, patients are more susceptible to recurrent lung infections and the development of bronchiectasis.[16–19] Additionally, chemotherapeutic agents used to treat these conditions often result in profound immunodeficiency (See "Medication that may cause immunodeficiency" slide).

Some medications which may cause immunodeficiency	
Anti convulsants	**Chemotherapeutic drugs**
Carbamazepine	Busulfan
Phenytoin	Cyclophosphamide
Valproate	Docetaxel
Anti hypertensives	Epirubicin
Amlodipine	Imatinib
Captopril	Melphalan
Enalapril	**NSAIDs**
Hydralazine	Diclofenac
Hydrochlorothiazide	Fenclofenac
Anti microbials	Meloxicam
Amphotericin B	Naproxen
Anti-virals (ie acyclovir, cidovir, foscarnet)	**Steroid-sparing Immunosuppressives**
Antimalarial agents (ie chloroquine)	Azathioprine
Cephalosporins/Penicillins	Cyclopsorine
Ethambutol	Gold salts
Tetracycline/Doxycycline	Mycophenolate mofetil
Biologics/Immunologicals	Penicillamine
Abatacept	Sirolimus
Alemtuzumab	Sulfasalazine
Belatacept	Tacrolimus
Certolizumab	**Other**
Muromonab	Glipizide
Rituximab	Gabapentin
Corticosteroids	Penicillamine
	Proton pump inhibitors (esomeprazole, lansoprazole, omperazole)
	Metoclopramide

HIV infection

The progression of disease in individuals infected with HIV varies greatly, but in most untreated patients, there is a progressive T-cell defect that results in a declining trend in CD4+ T-helper cell number. This declining trend may lead to decreased cellular immunity as well as T-cell–independent immunity, such as with local macrophage- and monocyte-dependent pulmonary immunity. Additionally, although most adult patients may have hypergammaglobulinemia with HIV infection, infants who are HIV positive can demonstrate severe hypogammaglobulinemia, suggesting that the development of humoral immunity is also affected.[20] Consequently, patients who are HIV positive are more prone to recurrent infections, both with usual and opportunistic pulmonary pathogens, including mycobacterium and S pneumonia.

Secondary Immunodeficiencies and Bronchiectasis

Reliable data regarding the relationship between secondary immune deficiencies and bronchiectasis are limited. Most of this data come from studies of patients with infectious complications caused by hematologic malignancy or the treatment of hematologic malignancy and patients who are HIV positive. It is generally regarded that other secondary causes of immunodeficiency do not result in a significant increased risk for recurrent pulmonary infection and bronchiectasis.

Hematological malignancies and bronchiectasis

A handful of case reports and series have described bronchiectasis complicating chemotherapy in acute myelogenous leukemia, CLL, multiple myeloma, and lymphomas. Multiple myeloma and CLL seem to be more commonly associated with bronchiectasis than the other hematologic malignancies, but there are no well-established incidence rates of bronchiectasis in patients with hematological malignancies. This lack may be caused by the combination of prolonged survival in patients with these malignancies and the higher frequency of secondary hypogammaglobulinemia in CLL and myeloma than in other hematologic disorders. It is suggested that patients with radiographic-proven bronchiectasis be assessed for hypogammaglobulinemia and considered for IVIG therapy. Bronchiectasis has also been reported, though less frequently, in acute hematological malignancies, perhaps as a consequence of severe lung infections or in the setting of profound immunodeficiency after chemotherapeutic intervention.[16,18,21]

Posttransplantation bronchiectasis

Hematopoietic stem cell transplantation (HSCT) is associated with an increased incidence of respiratory infections and prolonged defects in both cellular and humoral immunity in survivors.[22–26] These factors could predispose to bronchiectasis; in fact, serial CT scans after allograft HSCT can demonstrate rapidly developing bronchiectasis over a period of weeks to months. In addition, up to 10% of HSCT allograft recipients will develop bronchiolitis obliterans, which is the main pulmonary manifestation of graft-versus-host disease. This precedes the appearance of diffuse bronchiectasis in approximately 40% of cases.[27] Likewise, patients who develop bronchiolitis obliterans after lung transplantation may also have CT evidence of bronchiectasis, and there are cases of bronchiectasis developing after the transplantation of other solid organs, presumably because of impaired pulmonary immunity secondary to immunosuppressive therapy.[28]

HIV and bronchiectasis

The cause of HIV-related bronchiectasis is not well understood because of multiple confounding factors, such as concurrent pneumonia or tuberculosis; some studies also suggest an association of HIV in adults with an increase in chronic obstructive pulmonary disease. More reliable data may be from longitudinal pediatric studies. Up to 16% of children infected with HIV develop bronchiectasis.[20] Because of much better recent survival rates, the incidence of bronchiectasis in adults infected with HIV may also be significant. Bronchiectasis in children who are HIV positive is more likely in patients with CD4 counts less than 100 mm^3 or who have had recurrent pneumonia. Interestingly, there is also a specific association with lymphocytic interstitial pneumonitis (LIP), with up to 40% of HIV-infected children with LIP developing bronchiectasis.[29–31] There are no comparative data on the pattern and progression of bronchiectasis in patients who are HIV positive versus patients with bronchiectasis from other causes. More prevalence data and stratification of risk groups in HIV-positive patients are needed to direct recommendations for the management of bronchiectasis to prevent or slow the progression of lung disease.

Primary Immunodeficiencies

Primary immunodeficiencies are genetically predetermined disorders of the immune system, which result in decreased immunity and subsequent increase in susceptibility to infection. There are other diseases that result in recurrent or persistent infections, such as cystic fibrosis (CF) and ciliary dyskinesia, that also have a molecular genetic basis; these are discussed briefly but have generally not been thought to be predominantly driven by a functional defect within the immune system, although newer data suggest mucosal immunity is significantly diminished in these diseases. The molecular basis for about 70% to 80% of the more than 200 primary functional immune deficiencies that have been clinically described is known. For many of these diagnoses, the severity and spectrum of disease can vary widely. These conditions generally present during childhood, with about 70% of patients aged less than 20 years at the onset, with unusually frequent/recurrent infection or infection with uncommon organisms. Overall, about 60% of patients are male because many of the described disorders are X-linked. It is estimated that the incidence of symptomatic disease is about 1 out of 280 people.[32]

Primary immunodeficiencies are currently classified by the deficient immune system components involved, such as the B lymphocytes and immunoglobulins, T lymphocytes and natural killer (NK) cells, phagocytic cells, complement proteins, and receptor proteins, although there can be considerable overlap in immune function for these components, and combinations of deficiencies have been described in several clinical immunodeficiency diseases or syndromes.[32]

B lymphocyte disorders and hypogammaglobulinemia

It has been generally presumed that antibody deficiencies, which account for more than 50% of the described primary immunodeficiencies, result mostly from B-cell defects. Selective IgA deficiency is the most common B-cell disorder, and others are CVID and X-linked agammaglobulinemia (XLA). Patients with these diseases may have low or absent quantitative immunoglobulin isotypes and, in the case of CVID and XLA, low or absent specific antibody titers that can predispose them to infections with encapsulated gram-positive bacteria.

T lymphocyte disorders

Approximately 5% to 10% of primary immunodeficiencies are T-cell disorders. These diseases predispose patients to infection by viruses and opportunistic organisms, such as *Pneumocystis jiroveci* and fungi, as well as many common respiratory tract pathogens. Some T-cell disorders also cause immunoglobulin deficiencies because

B lymphocyte and T lymphocyte crosstalk is essential to generate specific antibodies. The more common T-cell disorders are DiGeorge syndrome, ZAP-70 deficiency, X-linked lymphoproliferative syndrome, and chronic mucocutaneous candidiasis.[33]

Disorders with combined B- and T-cell defects

Severe combined immunodeficiency (SCID) describes a set of disorders based on molecular defects affecting both B-cell and T-cell function. Several forms have been described and linked to specific genetic mutations, such as purine nucleoside phosphorylase deficiency. Immunoglobulin levels are normal or elevated with this deficiency, but because of inadequate T-cell function, antibody formation is impaired. Other genetic mutations identified in SCID include adenosine deaminase deficiency as well as mutations in the common gamma chain (encoded by the gene IL-2 receptor gamma), Janus kinase-3, and Artemis/DCLRE1C (which is essential to DNA repair).[34]

Disorders of innate immunity

Clinically significant primary NK cell defects are very rare and predispose patients to viral infections and tumors. Defects in the phagocytic and direct pathogen killing function of cells, such as macrophages, neutrophils, and monocytes, may account for 10% to 15% of described primary immunodeficiencies. Patients may have recurrent cutaneous staphylococcal and gram-negative infections. The most common phagocytic cell defects are chronic granulomatous disease (CGD), leukocyte adhesion deficiency, and Chédiak-Higashi syndrome.[32]

Complement deficiencies and more newly described toll-like receptor protein deficiencies are rare ($\leq$2% of described primary immunodeficiencies). Complement deficiencies can result in defective opsonization, phagocytosis, and lysis of pathogens, causing susceptibility to several bacteria. They can also cause defective clearance of antigen-antibody complexes, resulting in autoimmune inflammatory damage to an end-organ system (such as in lupus glomerulonephritis). Complement deficiency can also include the deficiency of C1 inhibitor, which underlies hereditary angioedema but is not associated with abnormal frequency or type of infections. C1 inhibitor deficiency is autosomal dominant, whereas the other complement deficiencies are autosomal recessive; the exception is properdin, which is X linked.[32]

The Relationship Between Immunodeficiency and Bronchiectasis

Infections as a cause for bronchiectasis in immunodeficiency

Almost all of the described immunodeficiencies and immunodeficiency syndromes can theoretically lead or contribute to bronchiectasis by increasing the risk of chronic or abnormally frequent and serious sinopulmonary infections. Overall, immunodeficiency is considered to be a rare cause of bronchiectasis in adults (0.5% to 2.4% versus 2% to 10% in the pediatric population).[5,35] However, some other reviewers have noted that of those presenting with bronchiectasis, as many as 7% of the adult population or one-third of the pediatric population have a primary immunodeficiency.[36] There are relatively few studies in the current literature that evaluate the incidence of immunodeficiency in patients with bronchiectasis, and most of these studies have been done at hospitals or academic centers specializing in respiratory diseases. Thus, the true incidence of immunodeficiency, especially particular immunodeficiencies, in patients with bronchiectasis is really unknown.

The pathophysiologic process leading to bronchiectasis is characterized by airway injury and dilation, which is then thought to promote the persistent colonization of pathogens in the affected bronchi as well as denude the airways of mucociliary structures that provide clearance of secretions. Common nasopharyngeal pathogens, such as *Streptococcus pneumoniae* and *Haemophilus influenzae*, infect both adults and children to cause acute bronchitis and pneumonia. It is speculated that impaired host immunity to these pathogens initiates the development of bronchiectasis, which then further compromises mucosal structures and immune defenses to permit infection and/or chronic colonization with environmental bacteria, such as with *Pseudomonas aeruginosa*.[36]

Because antibody-mediated immunity underlies the recognition of polysaccharide encapsulated respiratory pathogens, such as *S pneumoniae* and *H influenzae*, primary humoral immunodeficiency or antibody deficiency secondary to lymphoproliferative malignancies have been the most identified and studied in bronchiectasis patients. In one London hospital study, 122 out of 165 patients with radiographic evidence of bronchiectasis had an identifiable cause. Of those 122 patients, 11 had immunodeficiency compared with 17 with primary ciliary dyskinesia, 2 with cystic fibrosis, and 13 with allergic bronchopulmonary aspergillosis; the remaining majority of patients had a postinfectious cause or idiopathic bronchiectasis. Immunodeficiency in those 11 patients was diagnosed by low quantitative IgG levels as well as low postvaccination pneumococcal antibody titers, which characterize humoral immunodeficiency. Seven of these patients had common variable immunodeficiency with panhypogammaglobulinemia, and 4 patients had humoral immunodeficiency secondary to lymphoma or leukemia.[37]

Autoimmune or autoinflammatory disease as a cause for bronchiectasis in immunodeficiency

It is well accepted that certain systemic autoimmune diseases, such as rheumatoid arthritis (RA) and primary Sjögren disease, can lead to bronchiectasis. In an older study of 52 patients with a diagnosis of idiopathic bronchiectasis, there was a very high prevalence of rheumatoid factor (52%) and an increased prevalence of antinuclear factor (10%) in the patients with bronchiectasis compared with the control groups. The presence of these autoantibodies did not correlate closely with the severity of disease. Ten patients with bronchiectasis (19%) had one or more previously diagnosed autoimmune disorders; similarly, bronchiectasis was present in 2 out of 12 patients with recent-onset inflammatory RA.[38,39] In a more recent prospective series, HRCT demonstrated bronchiectasis in 6 out of 42 patients with autoantibody positivity for RA (positive anti-cyclic citrullinated peptide and/or 2 rheumatoid factor isotypes) but no inflammatory arthritis, and 2 of those patients then presented with frank RA within 13 months.[40–43] Reciprocally, it is well established that a significant number of patients with primary immunodeficiency, especially CVID, develop manifestations of autoimmunity. It is not clear whether the patients with RA and bronchiectasis have had significant infections or immunosuppression that contributed to their bronchiectasis,[44,45] or if there is an inflammatory phenomena independent from infection that underlies the mechanism for bronchiectasis in patients with immune dysregulation.

Humoral Immunodeficiencies Associated with Bronchiectasis

The development of humoral immunodeficiencies

There are multiple steps in B-cell differentiation and signal transmission that, if compromised, may lead to clinically significant antibody deficiency. Variable defects leading to a compromised antibody response to antigens result in CVID, which is actually a heterogeneous group of disorders with only a partially characterized molecular cause. A blockade in the maturation process from pre–B cell to immature B cell has been well characterized by a mutation in Bruton tyrosine kinase, which results in XLA. There have also been genetic mutations affecting the early pre–B-cell repertoire, such as with recombination-activating gene; this mutation also affects T-cell development and results in SCID. Defects in class switching and somatic hypermutation result in hyper IgM syndromes.

CVID

CVID is the second most common adult primary immunodeficiency (after selective IgA deficiency) and is characterized by low serum concentrations of IgG in combination with other isotypes, poor responses to immunizations, and recurrent sinopulmonary infections. The serum IgG level must be 2 standard deviations lower than normal. The underlying genetics of this heterogeneous group of disorders have only been partially described. About 10% to 20% of cases are familial; the first associated genes described have been inherited in an autosomal-dominant fashion, often with variable penetrance. Some of the more recently identified genetic defects associated with CVID have an autosomal recessive inheritance pattern. Of the 10% to 15% of patients with CVID who have had an underlying genetic abnormality described, most patients have defects in the transmembrane regulator, calcium modulator, and cyclophilin ligand interactor. Much smaller populations of people with CVID have had B- or T-cell anomalies related to surface receptors involved in crosstalk between the two sets of lymphocytes, such as with mutations of the inducible T-cell surface expressed CD28 costimulatory molecule and the B-cell activating factor receptor, which is the CD19 component of the coreceptor for the B-cell antigen receptor.[32]

This variety of mutations affecting the different components involved in the process of antibody production may also explain the diversity of clinical presentations and outcomes in patients with CVID. For example, as mentioned earlier, up to 25% to 30% of patients with CVID also develop autoimmune and/or lymphoproliferative sequelae, including inflammatory arthritis, colitis, lymphocytic lung disease, or granulomatous disease. These proinflammatory complications of immunodeficiency, thought to be caused by dysregulated immune cell signaling, may arguably contribute to the development of bronchiectasis independent of the problem of higher susceptibility to infection caused by the immunodeficiency.

The treatment of CVID with IVIG has been shown to both reduce the incidence of respiratory tract infections[46,47] and decrease inflammation associated with bronchiectasis.[48,49] Thus, early identification and treatment of CVID with IVIG may arguably improve prognostic outcomes associated with bronchiectasis. Traditionally, the dose of replacement IVIG given is based on keeping the IgG trough level, which often resulted in dosing that kept the trough at the lower end of the normal range. However, more recent studies have advocated that individualized dosing, based on infection end points in patients, may be needed to minimize the risk of bronchiectasis and chronic, progressive lung disease.[50]

XLA

Despite the absence of all antibody isotypes in agammaglobulinemia, the relative risk for patients with agammaglobulinemia of developing structural lung damage is reportedly less than patients with CVID.[51] XLA has been associated with up to 3% of cases of childhood bronchiectasis[39,52] but is only a rare cause in adults. No specific pattern of bronchiectasis in patients with XLA has clearly been described. The long-term prognosis has improved with aggressive treatment with IVIG and antibiotic therapy, although there are few data on the rate of progression of bronchiectasis, and chronic lung disease remains a significant cause of death.[53]

Selective IgA, IgM, and IgG subclass deficiencies

There are no clear data to support that isolated IgA, IgM, or IgG subclass deficiency is clinically relevant or if any specific chronic management or treatment is indicated. IgA deficiency is relatively common, with a prevalence of about 1 in 600. However, it is unlikely that, in the absence of concurrent IgG subclass deficiency or specific antibody deficiency, isolated IgA or IgM deficiency would lead to bronchiectasis and progressive lung disease.[54–56] However, IgG subclass deficiency, especially IgG2, has been associated with bronchiectasis in children.[57] However, because the incidence of IgG subclass deficiency in patients with bronchiectasis varies so greatly (anywhere from 4% to nearly 50%), the clinical significance of this correlative data is called into question. IgG subclass deficiency is a relatively common finding in the general population and may reflect transient, normal fluctuations in the immune system.[58] Nonetheless, it should be noted that IgG2 deficiency has been associated with low specific antibody responses to S pneumoniae or H influenzae bacteria that are associated with bronchiectasis.[59]

Specific antibody deficiency

In one small population study without matched controls, up to 58% of patients with idiopathic bronchiectasis were identified with specific antibody deficiency to polysaccharide antigens. This and other similar studies used the measurement of antibody titers to S pneumoniae and H influenzae after vaccination in comparison with the antibody response to protein antigen vaccination, such as tetanus or diphtheria, to identify patients with specific antibody deficiency to these polysaccharide-encapsulated organisms; the lower-limit threshold to define the criteria for this immunodeficiency has been frequently debated, and there is still no clear consensus.[59] Antibody responses to vaccination with polysaccharide antigens are variable and affected by age, and up to 10% of the normal population may be nonresponders.[60–62] A larger series of adult patients with bronchiectasis suggest specific antibody deficiency has an incidence varying from 4% to 11%.[60,63–65] An impaired specific antibody response was associated with selected IgG subclass deficiencies in some patients.[57] It is clear that higher-powered, control-matched studies are needed to evaluate any relationship between specific antibody deficiency and bronchiectasis.

Other Primary Immunodeficiencies and Bronchiectasis

Transporter antigen peptide deficiency syndrome

Transporter antigen peptide (TAP) proteins are required for the transfer of peptide antigens from the cytosol into the endoplasmic reticulum, where they associate with human leukocyte antigen (HLA)-1 for presentation on cell surfaces. Autosomal recessive mutations in the TAP1 or TAP2 genes result in reduced HLA-1 expression and CD8 lymphocyte numbers but increased NK and $\gamma\delta$ T cells.[36,66,67] Most patients with TAP deficiency have recurrent sinopulmonary infections with common respiratory tract bacterial pathogens and develop bronchiectasis.[66,67] Only a handful of families with TAP deficiency have been described, and this genetic defect will be responsible for a vanishingly small proportion of cases of bronchiectasis. However, the association of TAP deficiency and other very rare familial T-cell disorders with bronchiectasis[68–70] demonstrates that there are previously unsuspected mechanisms of immunity to extracellular bacterial pathogens involving CD8 lymphocytes that require further investigation. In addition, it has been suggested that an excess of NK and $\gamma\delta$ T cells might promote bronchiectasis because of a dysregulated inflammatory response to infection with bacterial pathogens.

Macrophage or neutrophil functional deficiencies

There have been many inherited disorders affecting neutrophil function described, such as CGD, leukocyte adhesion deficiency, and Chédiak-Higashi syndrome. Although these disorders are extremely rare, making it difficult to accurately evaluate their clinical associations, neutrophil disorders classically lead to recurrent pneumonia. In a relatively large series of adult patients with bronchiectasis, tests of neutrophil function, such as flow cytometry for DHR, could only occasionally identify patients with abnormal responses. Even in these patients, the relationship of the defect to bronchiectasis is not clear. CGD has been associated with cases of bronchiectasis in some pediatric case reports, but these reports have significant selection bias. There is only a weak association of neutrophil defects with bronchiectasis and this may be attributable to the fact that the range of pathogens these patients are most susceptible to includes *Staphylococcus aureus*, *Nocardia*, *Aspergillus*, and *Candida* species but excludes *S pneumoniae* and *H influenzae*, which are the pathogens most closely associated with development of bronchiectasis.[52,71,72]

Primary defects of macrophage function generally affect intracellular killing and lead to increased incidences of infection with intracellular pathogens (such as mycobacteria, *Histoplasma*, *Listeria*, and *Salmonella* species) and have not been associated with the development of bronchiectasis. The extent to which functional polymorphisms of phagocytic receptors, such as Fc gamma RIIA H/R 131, or pattern recognition receptors, such as toll-like receptors, may predispose to bronchiectasis is unclear.[71,72]

Hyper IgE syndrome

Hyper IgE syndrome (Job syndrome) is a rare autosomal-dominant inherited syndrome that causes susceptibility to a range of infections and presents with a characteristic set of bone, dental, vascular, and joint abnormalities. Most patients have the classic clinical triad of extremely high elevations in serum IgE levels, recurrent pneumonias, and soft tissue abscesses.[32,36] Patients have impaired T-helper cell type 17 (Th17) CD4 response, which has a role in mucosal immunity to some respiratory pathogens, such as *Klebsiella pneumoniae* and *S pneumoniae*, as well as *S aureus* and *Candida*. Th17 CD4 immune responses aid in neutrophil recruitment to sites of infection and to the local mucosal communities. Pneumonias in patients with hyper IgE syndrome can be complicated by pneumatoceles but can also lead to bronchiectasis in a significant proportion of patients.[73–79]

Inherited disorders of DNA repair

Ataxia telangiectasia, an inherited disorder of DNA repair, and Wiskott-Aldrich syndrome, an X-linked immunodeficiency caused by mutations in the WASP gene, increase the risk of infections by affecting the development of adaptive immunity. Many of these patients are antibody deficient and have bronchiectasis.[80] Mutations in the WASP gene can result in low levels of T and B lymphocytes, NK cells, and serum IgM. Patients subsequently tend to develop infections with encapsulated organisms and therefore are at risk of bronchiectasis.[81] Both of these disorders are rare causes of bronchiectasis in pediatric case series.[52,72]

Complement deficiency found in patients with bronchiectasis

Immunity to extracellular bacterial pathogens relies on the complement system; thus, it is not surprising that inherited complement deficiencies, such as C2 or mannose-binding lectin (MBL) deficiency, have been associated with recurrent respiratory infections. As a consequence, there are reports of MBL deficiency isolated in patients with bronchiectasis; however, it should be noted that MBL deficiency figures to be a relatively common condition, affecting up to 25% of the population, and the reports of bronchiectasis with this condition are quite rare. It is speculated that concurrent MBL deficiency in patients with CVID and CF may increase the incidence and severity of bronchiectasis. Lower levels of L-ficolin, another MBL pathway opsonin, has also been found in patients with bronchiectasis compared with controls, but those data have not been replicated. Other complement deficiencies are very rare, and there are no data on these deficiencies and bronchiectasis.[36]

Cystic fibrosis and ciliary dyskinesia

Patients with CF and ciliary dyskinesia will likely develop bronchiectasis caused by persistently poor mucociliary clearance. Neither had been thought to be true genetic defects of the immune system. However, more recent data suggest mutations of the CF transmembrane conductance regulator in CF also cause a variety of defects in immune cell function involved in mucosal innate immunity. Studies have demonstrated impaired phagocyte function, reduced efficacy of antibacterial peptides, failure of bacterial internalization by epithelial cells, and an exaggerated inflammatory response to infection. Aside from a problem with mucociliary clearance, multiple defects in innate immunity could play a significant role in the development of bronchiectasis in patients with CF, but further research is required.[82]

Causes of hypogammaglobulinemia	
Non Malignant Systemic Conditions	**Infectious Diseases**
Immunodeficiency caused by hypercatabolism of immunoglobulin	HIV
	Congenital Rubella
Immunodeficiency caused by excessive loss of immunoglobulins (nephrosis, severe burns, lymphangiectasia, severe diarrhea)	Congenital infection with CMV
	Congenital infection with Toxoplasma gondii
Genetic Disorders (Other than CVID)	
	Epstein-Barr Virus
Ataxia Telangiectasia	**Malignancy**
Autosomal forms of SCID	Chronic Lymphocytic Leukemia
Hyper IgM Immunodeficiency	Immunodeficiency with Thymoma
Transcobalamin II deficiency	Non Hodgkin's lymphoma
X-linked agammaglobulinemia	B cell malignancy
X-linked lymphoproliferative disorder (EBV associated)	Myelofibrosis
X-linked SCID	Metastatic solid cancers (brain, lung, intestinal)
Some metabolic disorders	**Medications**
Chromosomal Anomalies	Antimalarial agents
Chromosome 18q- Syndrome	Captopril
Monosomy 22	Carbamazepine
Trisomy 8	Glucocorticoids
Trisomy 21	Fenclofenac
	Gold salts
	Penicillamine
	Phenytoin
	Sulfasalazine
	Rituximab

Suggested Immunologic Evaluation of Patients with Bronchiectasis

The identity of the infecting organisms are of most value to direct laboratory investigations; encapsulated bacteria suggest B-cell immunodeficiencies; fungi, viruses, and mycobacteria usually present in T-cell immunodeficiencies; and catalase-positive organisms (eg, *Staphylococcus, Aspergillus*) suggest a neutrophil dysfunction. Generally, a sequential approach to investigating immune function in patients with bronchiectasis or recurrent infections is recommended. Initial measurements of total serum Ig, IgG subclasses, specific antibody levels before and after vaccination (See Secondary Causes of Hypogammabulinemia slide) should be performed, secondary causes of hypogammaglobulinemia should be considered, as well as HIV testing if there is clinical indication. Further testing and referral to an immunologist may then be considered; additional evaluation may include tests to evaluate cellular function (such as T- and B-cell immunophenotyping) and innate immunity (such as neutrophil superoxide measurements (CGD) and complement). Lastly, gene sequencing and functional assays may be considered.[32,36]

Relationship Between Immunodeficiency, Bronchiectasis, and Asthma

In summary, the concomitant presence of immunodeficiency in patients with existing asthma and chronic airway obstruction increases susceptibility to recurrent or persistent infections and/or airway inflammation. This susceptibility may drive the process of bronchiectasis and result in increased airway secretions, thereby further increasing the risk for pulmonary infection. This promotes a cycle of airway inflammation, bronchial obstruction, and poorly controlled asthma. There is a high incidence of bronchiectasis in patients with severe asthma, although the precise frequency of bronchiectasis causing asthma is unclear, as both asthma and irreversible airway obstruction can also be complications of chronic bronchiectasis due to persistent bronchial wall inflammation. In patients with bronchiectasis, if humoral immunodeficiency such as CVID is identified and treated with IVIG, there is a reduction in frequency and severity of pulmonary infections. Better control of infection risk in patients with immunodeficiency and bronchiectasis will lead to better control of asthma and potentially prevent or mitigate chronic lung disease sequelae caused by both uncontrolled asthma and progressive bronchiectasis.

REFERENCES

1. Barker AF. Clinical manifestations and diagnosis of bronchiectasis in adults. UpToDate; 2012.
2. Bisaccioni C, Aun MV, Cajuela E, et al. Comorbidities in severe asthma: frequency of rhinitis, nasal polyposis, gastroesophageal reflux disease, vocal cord dysfunction and bronchiectasis. Clinics (Sao Paulo) 2009;64(8):769–73.
3. Boyton RJ, Smith J, Ward R, et al. HLA-C and killer cell immunoglobulin-like receptor genes in idiopathic bronchiectasis. Am J Respir Crit Care Med 2006; 173:327–33.
4. Boyton RJ, Smith J, Jones M, et al. Human leucocyte antigen class II association in idiopathic bronchiectasis, a disease of chronic lung infection, implicates a role for adaptive immunity. Clin Exp Immunol 2008;152:95–101.
5. Oguzulgen IK, Kervan F, Ozis T, et al. The impact of bronchiectasis in clinical presentation of asthma. South Med J 2007;100(5):468–71.
6. Haidopoulou K, Calder A, Jones A, et al. Bronchiectasis secondary to primary immunodeficiency in children: longitudinal changes in structure and function. Pediatr Pulmonol 2009;44(7):669–75.

7. Klemola T. Deficiency of immunoglobulin A. Ann Clin Res 1987;19:248–57.
8. Szczawinska-Poplonyk A. An overlapping syndrome of allergy and immune deficiency in children. J Allergy (Cairo) 2012;2012:658279 [E-Review article].
9. Taylor AE, Finney-Hayward TK, Quint JK, et al. Defective macrophage phagocytosis of bacteria in COPD. Eur Respir J 2010;35:1039–47.
10. Tanawuttiwat T, Harindhanavudhi T. Bronchiectasis: pulmonary manifestation in chronic graft versus host disease after bone marrow transplantation. Am J Med Sci 2009;337:292.
11. Shabestari MS, Rezaei N. Asthma and allergic rhinitis in a patient with BTK deficiency. J Investig Allergol Clin Immunol 2008;18(4):300–4.
12. Ogershok PR, Hogan MB, Welch JE, et al. Spectrum of illness in pediatric common variable immunodeficiency. Ann Allergy Asthma Immunol 2006;97(5): 653–6.
13. Agondi RC, Barros MT, Rizzo LV, et al. Allergic asthma in patients with common variable immunodeficiency. Allergy 2010;65(4):510–5.
14. Amorosa JK, Miller RW, Laraya-Cuasay L, et al. Bronchiectasis in children with lymphocytic interstitial pneumonia and acquired immune deficiency syndrome. Plain film and CT observations. Pediatr Radiol 1992;22:603–6.
15. Corominas M, Garcia JF, Mestre M, et al. Predictors of atopy in HIV-infected patients. Ann Allergy Asthma Immunol 2000;84(6):607–11.
16. Kearney PJ, Kershaw CR, Stevenson PA. Bronchiectasis in acute leukaemia. Br Med J 1977;2:857–9.
17. Kilpatrick DC, Chalmers JD, MacDonald SL, et al. Stable bronchiectasis is associated with low serum L-ficolin concentrations. Clin Respir J 2009;3:29–33.
18. Knowles GK, Stanhope R, Green M. Bronchiectasis complicating chronic lymphatic leukaemia with hypogammaglobulinaemia. Thorax 1980;35:217–8.
19. Lambrecht BN, Neyt K, GeurtsvanKessel CH. Pulmonary defense mechanisms and inflammatory pathways in bronchiectasis. Eur Respir Mon 2011;52:11–21.
20. Love JT Jr, Shearer WT. Hypogammaglobulinemia in HIV-infected infants. N Engl J Med 1995;333(5):321–2.
21. Okada F, Ando Y, Kondo Y, et al. Thoracic CT findings of adult T-cell leukemia or lymphoma. AJR Am J Roentgenol 2004;182:761–7.
22. Morehead RS. Bronchiectasis in bone marrow transplantation. Thorax 1997;52: 392–3.
23. Parkman R. Antigen-specific immunity following hematopoietic stem cell transplantation. Blood Cells Mol Dis 2008;40:91–3.
24. Paganin F, Seneterre E, Chanez P, et al. Computed tomography of the lungs in asthma: influence of disease severity and etiology. Am J Respir Crit Care Med 1996;153:110–4.
25. Patel IS, Vlahos I, Wilkinson TM, et al. Bronchiectasis, exacerbation indices, and inflammation in chronic obstructive pulmonary disease. Am J Respir Crit Care Med 2004;170:400–7.
26. Pasteur MC, Helliwell SM, Houghton SJ, et al. An investigation into causative factors in patients with bronchiectasis. Am J Respir Crit Care Med 2000;162: 1277–84.
27. Gunn ML, Godwin JD, Kanne JP, et al. High-resolution CT findings of bronchiolitis obliterans syndrome after hematopoietic stem cell transplantation. J Thorac Imaging 2008;23:244–50.
28. de Jong PA, Dodd JD, Coxson HO, et al. Bronchiolitis obliterans following lung transplantation: early detection using computed tomographic scanning. Thorax 2006;61:799–804.

29. Baris S, Ercan H, Cagan HH, et al. Efficacy of intravenous immunoglobulin treatment in children with common variable immunodeficiency. J Investig Allergol Clin Immunol 2011;21(7):514–21.
30. Berman DM, Mafut D, Djokic B, et al. Risk factors for the development of bronchiectasis in HIV-infected children. Pediatr Pulmonol 2007;42:871–5.
31. Sheikh S, Madiraju K, Steiner P, et al. Bronchiectasis in pediatric AIDS. Chest 1997;112:1202–7.
32. Buckley RH. Overview of immunodeficiency disorder. Merck manual. 2008.
33. Buckley RH. Primary immunodeficiency diseases due to defects in lymphocytes. N Engl J Med 2000;343:1313–24.
34. Yee A, De Ravin SS, Elliott E, et al. Severe combined immunodeficiency: a national surveillance study. Pediatr Allergy Immunol 2008;19(4):298–302.
35. Bilton D, Jones AL. Bronchiectasis: epidemiology and causes. Eur Respir Mon 2011;52:1–10.
36. Brown JS, Baxendale H, Floto RA. Immunodeficiencies associated with bronchiectasis. Eur Respir Mon 2011;52:178–91.
37. Shoemark A, Ozerovitch L, Wilson R. Aetiology in adult patients with bronchiectasis. Respir Med 2007;101:1161–70.
38. Hilton AM, Doyle L. Immunological abnormalities in bronchiectasis with chronic bronchial suppuration. Br J Dis Chest 1978;72(3):207–16.
39. Lieberman-Maran L, Orzano IM, Passero MA, et al. Bronchiectasis in rheumatoid arthritis: report of four cases and a review of the literature–implications for management with biologic response modifiers. Semin Arthritis Rheum 2006;35:379–87.
40. Demoruelle MK, Weisman MH, Simonian PL, et al. Brief report: airways abnormalities and rheumatoid arthritis-related autoantibodies in subjects without arthritis: early injury or initiating site of autoimmunity? Arthritis Rheum 2012;64(6):1756–61.
41. Dhasmana DJ, Wilson R. Bronchiectasis and autoimmune disease. Eur Respir Mon 2011;52:192–210.
42. Dogru D, Ozbas Gerceker F, Yalcin E, et al. The role of TAP1 and TAP2 gene polymorphism in idiopathic bronchiectasis in children. Pediatr Pulmonol 2007;42:237–41.
43. Doring G, Gulbins E. Cystic fibrosis and innate immunity: how chloride channel mutations provoke lung disease. Cell Microbiol 2009;11:208–16.
44. Cooper N, Arnold DM. The effect of rituximab on humoral and cell mediated immunity and infection in the treatment of autoimmune disease. Br J Haematol 2010;149:3–13.
45. Cooper N, Davies EG, Thrasher AJ. Repeated courses of rituximab for autoimmune cytopenias may precipitate profound hypogammaglobulinaemia requiring replacement intravenous immunoglobulin. Br J Haematol 2009;146:120–2.
46. Busse PJ, Razvi S, Cunningham-Rundles C. Efficacy of intravenous immunoglobulin in the prevention of pneumonia in patients with common variable immunodeficiency. J Allergy Clin Immunol 2002;109:1001–4.
47. Casanova JL, Abel L. Human genetics of infectious diseases: a unified theory. EMBO J 2007;26:915–22.
48. Eijkhout HW, van Der Meer JW, Kallenberg CG, et al. The effect of two different dosages of intravenous immunoglobulin on the incidence of recurrent infections in patients with primary hypogammaglobulinemia. A randomized, double-blind, multicenter crossover trial. Ann Intern Med 2001;135:165–74.

49. Eisen DP. Mannose-binding lectin deficiency and respiratory tract infection. J Innate Immun 2010;2:114–22.
50. Lucas M, Lee M, Lortan J, et al. Infection outcomes in patients with common variable immunodeficiency disorders: relationship to immunoglobulin therapy over 22 years. J Allergy Clin Immunol 2010;125:1354–60.
51. Aghamohammadi A, Allahverdi A, Abolhassani H, et al. Comparison of pulmonary diseases in common variable immunodeficiency and X-linked agammaglobulinaemia. Respirology 2010;15:289–95.
52. Li AM, Sonnappa S, Lex C, et al. Non-CF bronchiectasis: does knowing the aetiology lead to changes in management? Eur Respir J 2005;26:8–14.
53. Howard V, Greene JM, Pahwa S, et al. The health status and quality of life of adults with X-linked agammaglobulinemia. Clin Immunol 2006;118:201–8.
54. Jeurissen A, Bossuyt X, Snapper CM. T cell-dependent and -independent responses. J Immunol 2004;172:2728.
55. Jonsson G, Truedsson L, Sturfelt G, et al. Hereditary C2 deficiency in Sweden: frequent occurrence of invasive infection, atherosclerosis, and rheumatic disease. Medicine (Baltimore) 2005;84:23–34.
56. Stead A, Douglas JG, Broadfoot CJ, et al. Humoral immunity and bronchiectasis. Clin Exp Immunol 2002;130:325–30.
57. Umetsu DT, Ambrosino DM, Quinti I, et al. Recurrent sinopulmonary infection and impaired antibody response to bacterial capsular polysaccharide antigen in children with selective IgG-subclass deficiency. N Engl J Med 1985;313:1247–51.
58. Nahm MH, Macke K, Kwon OH, et al. Immunologic and clinical status of blood donors with subnormal levels of IgG2. J Allergy Clin Immunol 1990;85:769–77.
59. van Kessel DA, van Velzen-Blad H, van den Bosch JMM, et al. Impaired pneumococcal antibody response in bronchiectasis of unknown aetiology. Eur Respir J 2005;25:482–9.
60. Go ES, Ballas ZK. Anti-pneumococcal antibody response in normal subjects: a meta-analysis. J Allergy Clin Immunol 1996;98:205–15.
61. Gregersen S, Aalokken TM, Mynarek G, et al. Development of pulmonary abnormalities in patients with common variable immunodeficiency: associations with clinical and immunologic factors. Ann Allergy Asthma Immunol 2010;104:503–10.
62. Rodrigo MJ, Miravitlles M, Cruz MJ, et al. Characterization of specific immunoglobulin G (IgG) and its subclasses (IgG1 and IgG2) against the 23-valent pneumococcal vaccine in a healthy adult population: proposal for response criteria. Clin Diagn Lab Immunol 1997;4:168–72.
63. Lipsitch M, Whitney CG, Zell E, et al. Are anticapsular antibodies the primary mechanism of protection against invasive pneumococcal disease? PLoS Med 2005;2:e15.
64. Litzman J, Freiberger T, Grimbacher B, et al. Mannose-binding lectin gene polymorphic variants predispose to the development of bronchopulmonary complications but have no influence on other clinical and laboratory symptoms or signs of common variable immunodeficiency. Clin Exp Immunol 2008;153:324–30.
65. Miravitlles M, Vendrell M, de Gracia J. Antibody deficiency in bronchiectasis. Eur Respir J 2005;26:178–80.
66. Gadola SD, Moins-Teisserenc HT, Trowsdale J, et al. TAP deficiency syndrome. Clin Exp Immunol 2000;121:173–8.
67. Zimmer J, Andres E, Donato L, et al. Clinical and immunological aspects of HLA class I deficiency. QJM 2005;98:719–27.

68. Chatila T, Wong R, Young M, et al. An immunodeficiency characterized by defective signal transduction in T lymphocytes. N Engl J Med 1989;320:696–702.
69. Contoli M, Message SD, Laza-Stanca V, et al. Role of deficient type III interferon-lambda production in asthma exacerbations. Nat Med 2006;12:1023–6.
70. Crothers K, Butt AA, Gibert CL, et al. Increased COPD among HIV-positive compared to HIV-negative veterans. Chest 2006;130:1326–33.
71. Andrews T, Sullivan KE. Infections in patients with inherited defects in phagocytic function. Clin Microbiol Rev 2003;16:597–621.
72. Nikolaizik WH, Warner JO. Aetiology of chronic suppurative lung disease. Arch Dis Child 1994;70:141–2.
73. Aujla SJ, Dubin PJ, Kolls JK. Th17 cells and mucosal host defense. Semin Immunol 2007;19:377–82.
74. Holland SM, DeLeo FR, Elloumi HZ, et al. STAT3 mutations in the hyper-IgE syndrome. N Engl J Med 2007;357:1608–19.
75. Holmes AH, Pelton S, Steinbach S, et al. HIV related bronchiectasis. Thorax 1995; 50:1227.
76. Holmes AH, Trotman-Dickenson B, Edwards A, et al. Bronchiectasis in HIV disease. Q J Med 1992;85:875–82.
77. Paulson ML, Freeman AF, Holland SM. Hyper IgE syndrome: an update on clinical aspects and the role of signal transducer and activator of transcription 3. Curr Opin Allergy Clin Immunol 2008;8:527–33.
78. Pijnenburg MW, Cransberg K, Wolff E, et al. Bronchiectasis in children after renal or liver transplantation: a report of five cases. Pediatr Transplant 2004;8:71–4.
79. Zhang Z, Clarke TB, Weiser JN. Cellular effectors mediating Th17-dependent clearance of pneumococcal colonization in mice. J Clin Invest 2009;119:1899–909.
80. Bott. 2007.
81. Ochs HD, Filipovich AH, Veys P, et al. Wiskott-Aldrich syndrome: diagnosis, clinical and laboratory manifestations, and treatment. Biol Blood Marrow Transplant 2009;15:84–90.
82. Moskwa P, Lorentzen D, Excoffon KJ, et al. A novel host defense system of airways is defective in cystic fibrosis. Am J Respir Crit Care Med 2007;175:174–83.

RADS and Its Variants
Asthma by Another Name

Annyce Mayer, MD, MSPH[a,b,]*, Karin Pacheco, MD, MSPH[a,b]

KEYWORDS

- Reactive airways dysfunction syndrome • Work-exacerbated asthma
- Irritant exposures • Irritant asthma

KEY POINTS

- Acute high-level irritant exposures can cause asthma and exacerbate underlying asthma.
- Lower-level irritant exposures can at least exacerbate underlying asthma, although there is emerging consensus that recurrent lower-level exposures may also cause asthma.
- There is overlap between the exposures that have caused acute irritant-induced asthma and work-exacerbated asthma (WEA), many of which are also sensitizers.
- New-onset asthma in workers following lower-level irritant exposures, with no prior history of respiratory symptoms or asthma, may well be limited to a subset of "susceptible" hosts, such as those with asymptomatic airway hyperresponsiveness, atopy, and those who "outgrew" childhood asthma.
- The ATS statement on WEA has identified research needs to better define risk factors, biologic mechanisms, and outcomes in WEA, which should help facilitate necessary interventions in the medical system, as well as to formulate and apply strategies for prevention.

INTRODUCTION

Asthma is a chronic respiratory condition characterized by variable airflow obstruction, airways hyperresponsiveness, and airway inflammation. Approximately 7.7% of US adults of working age have asthma[1] and an estimated 16.3% of all cases of adult asthma have been attributed to asthma caused or exacerbated by workplace exposures.[2] Many other conditions and factors, such as rhinosinusitis, gastroesophageal reflux disease (GERD), vocal cord dysfunction, and cigarette smoking, may trigger symptoms that mimic asthma but are not, and these are covered elsewhere in this issue. Other, more serious conditions that mimic asthma include hypersensitivity

---

[a] Division of Environmental and Occupational Health Sciences, Department of Medicine, National Jewish Health, 1400 Jackson Street, Denver, CO 80206, USA; [b] Department of Environmental/Occupational Health, Colorado School of Public Health - University of Colorado Denver, 13001 E. 17th Place, B119, Bldg. 500, 3rd Floor, Aurora, CO 80045, USA
* Corresponding author.
E-mail address: mayera@njhealth.org

Immunol Allergy Clin N Am 33 (2013) 79–93
http://dx.doi.org/10.1016/j.iac.2012.10.011
0889-8561/13/$ – see front matter © 2013 Elsevier Inc. All rights reserved.

pneumonitis, which can be caused by low molecular weight irritants that are also sensitizers,[3–6] bronchiolitis obliterans,[7,8] and irritant/odorant-triggered cough.[9–11] Whereas asthma caused by sensitization is well described and well accepted,[12–16] it is not the primary focus of this article. On the other hand, reactive airways dysfunction syndrome (RADS) and other variants of irritant-induced or irritant-exacerbated asthma may not always initially appear as asthma, but are, in fact, alternate presentations of asthma. Therefore, occupational and environmental exposures that can cause or exacerbate asthma should be considered as well. Although unique conditions exist in the workplace that more often lead to the type of exposures that can cause or exacerbate asthma, exposure to sensitizers and irritants that exacerbate or cause asthma can also occur in the home, during avocational activities, and following accidental industrial releases into the environment. Thus, although the terms occupational and workplace are used in this article, environmental sources of these exposures should also be considered.

The role of irritants in the causation of asthma is now well established. RADS was originally defined in 1981 by Brooks and Lockey[17] and detailed in case series of new-onset asthma syndrome within 24 hours following a single, high-level irritant exposure.[18] Since that time, modifications to the case definition have been proposed, and more recently the term "acute irritant asthma" has been used, with good consensus that this is not just an asthma syndrome but indeed occupational asthma.[14,16,19,20] Asthma has been reported after lower-level irritant exposures, with considerable controversy regarding whether or not the lower-level irritant exposure caused the asthma,[21,22] was a result of concurrent immunologic sensitization,[16,23] or caused an exacerbation of underlying asthma.[14–16,24,25] Work-exacerbated asthma (WEA) is defined as "preexisting or concurrent asthma that is worsened by workplace conditions,"[25] in which there is a temporal association between asthma exacerbations and work in a place where conditions exist that can exacerbate asthma, but that asthma caused by work (immunologic asthma and acute irritant asthma) is considered unlikely. WEA is often not compensable under workers' compensation.

This article covers the different clinical variants of irritant-induced asthma, specifically focusing on high level irritant-induced asthma and irritant-induced WEA reviews known causes, addresses the often adverse medical and socioeconomic outcomes of this complex condition, and considers issues of causation from an occupational and environmental medicine perspective.

CLINICAL VIGNETTE 1

John Adams is a 45-year-old city maintenance worker. He is a never-smoker and has no history of asthma or other medical problems. He performs maintenance inside city facilities, including the wastewater treatment plant. On one occasion, a regulator malfunction caused the sudden high-pressure release of 100% chlorine into the very small room where he was working. The sudden release caused him to take in a deep breath, and he experienced immediate cough, burning eyes and nose, chest burning and tightness, and shortness of breath. He was taken to the emergency department and placed on oxygen. He is not sure about what other treatment he received, but after a period of time he felt somewhat better and was discharged. Most of his symptoms continued to improve, but the dry cough persisted. He noted chest tightness and shortness of breath with exertion, such as walking in the mountains. His chest symptoms were also triggered by irritants, such as cigarette smoke, perfume, and dust, which had never bothered him before. He seeks medical attention for these symptoms 3 months later. Could this be asthma?

ACUTE IRRITANT ASTHMA

Yes, asthma should be considered as part of the differential diagnosis, and should be confirmed by methacholine challenge or bronchodilator responsiveness. The presentation is consistent with RADS, defined as asthma caused by a single, high level, irritant exposure hypothesized to cause acute bronchial mucosal damage leading to airways hyperresponsiveness. Whereas allergen exposures are well-documented causes of asthma, the role of irritants in the causation of asthma has been recognized only more recently. RADS was originally described as a "persistent asthma syndrome" after high-level irritant exposure.[17,18] Brooks noted that although the illness clinically simulated bronchial asthma and was associated with airways hyperreactivity, it differed from typical occupational asthma because of rapid onset (within 24 hours) after a single high-level environmental exposure, and this period of time is too short for the development of sensitization.[18] Although the validity of the syndrome as new-onset asthma was initially debated,[26,27] numerous case reports have followed,[9,28–32] and it is now widely accepted that acute high-level irritant exposures not only cause a syndrome that mimics asthma but can cause asthma itself.[14–16,19,20] Tarlo and Broder introduced the term "irritant-induced asthma" in 1989 to include workers in their case series who had high-level irritant exposure on more than one occasion,[33] which has been subsequently reported by others.[30] Other studies included those with onset of symptoms up to 7 days after a well-defined spill; they identified additional cases that otherwise met the case definition.[34] The term "acute irritant-induced asthma" was recently proposed,[16,20] and for workers without any prior history of asthma, the term is an accurate unifying descriptor. A list of some of the exposures reported to have caused acute irritant asthma, termed RADS and asthma after spills or accidental exposures, are shown in **Table 1**. The clinical criteria for RADS described by Brooks[18] and modifications that have been proposed are shown in **Box 1**.

In many cases, the symptoms resolve within months, but they can persist in some.[9,18,29–32,35,36] The long-term sequelae can be significant. One long-term follow-up study of workers (52% participation) with claims accepted by the workers' compensation agency in Quebec revealed significant ongoing respiratory impairment and psychosocial impact two years after initial symptoms. These patients presented with acute irritant-induced asthma due to a well-defined high-level accidental release (57% chlorine) and had symptoms that developed within 24 hours and persisted beyond 3 months. All subjects still had respiratory symptoms; 68% were on inhaled corticosteroids, there had been no significant improvement in forced expiratory volume in 1 second (FEV1) (mean FEV1 74.5% ± 19.5% predicted), and most still demonstrated airways hyperresponsiveness based on methacholine challenge or improvement after bronchodilator. There was a negative impact on quality of life, and about one-third had abnormal depression scores.[37] The long-term impact was similar to that reported in immunologic asthma.[38]

CLINICAL VIGNETTE 2

Michael Janvier is a 54-year-old insulator in a large plant. He has a 5-pack-year history and had stopped smoking at age 30. He has no prior history of respiratory symptoms. He has performed installation, repair, and routine maintenance on the pipes in a chrome-plating shop on and off over the past 10 years. Some of the pipes were located 4 to 5 feet above the acid baths. Depending on the job, he could spend several weeks or even months at a time in that shop. He sometimes felt burning in his eyes, nose, and throat, as well as some cough, although these symptoms were fairly mild and typically resolved later that evening or the next day. About a year ago, he began

Table 1
Reported high-level irritant exposures associated with development of acute irritant-induced asthma, along with pH, potential for thermal injury, and sensitizer potential

Author	Outcome	Reported Chemical	High or Low pH	Potential for Thermal Injury	Potential Sensitizer
Brooks et al,[18] 1985	RADS after single high-level exposure	Uranium hexafluoride			−
		Floor sealant			?
		Spray paint (3)			?
		35% hydrazine			
		Heated acid	+	+	
		Fumigating fog			?
		Metal coat remover	?		
		Fire/smoke		+	?
Tarlo and Broder,[33] 1989	RADS after 1 or more high-level exposures	Acids	+		
		Calcium oxide			
		Chlorine, sulfuric acid, sulfur dioxide	+		
		HCl, phosgene	+		
		Calcium oxide, welding fumes			?
		Burnt paint fumes		?	?
		Spray paint no isocyanate			
		Chlorine			
		Toluene diisocyanate			+
		Diphenyl methane diisocyanate			+
Chatkin et al,[45] 2007	Asthma after spills or accidental exposures	Isocyanates			+
		Paint			?
		Solvents			
		Chlorine			
		Ammonia	+		
		Calcium oxide	+		
		Acrylates			+
		Amines			+
		Epoxy resins			+
		Dyes			?
		Ozone			?
		Pesticides			
		Wood dust			?
		Methylmercaptan			

The "+" refers to the listed chemical exposures that have one or more of the other properties: high or low pH, potential for thermal injury and/or are potential sensitizers. The "?" refers to those chemical exposures that might have one of those properties, but there is insufficient information about the exposure to determine.
   Abbreviation: RADS, reactive airways dysfunction syndrome.

to notice worsening shortness of breath while running and playing soccer. He also started awakening at night with chest tightness about once a week. A cardiac evaluation was negative, including a normal stress echocardiogram. His symptoms continue to worsen and he seeks further medical attention. Could this be this asthma?

ASTHMA FOLLOWING LOWER-LEVEL IRRITANT EXPOSURES

In 2005, Brooks[39] introduced the term "not-so-sudden onset" irritant-induced asthma to describe the exposures in a subgroup of subjects who had onset of asthma

---

Box 1
Clinical criteria for acute irritant-induced asthma[a]

1. A documented absence of preceding respiratory complaints.

2. The onset of symptoms occurred after 1 or more high-level exposures.[b]

3. The exposure was to a gas, smoke, fume, or vapor that was present in very high concentrations and had irritant qualities to its nature.

4. The onset of symptoms occurred within 24 hours[c] after the exposure and persisted for at least 3 months.

5. Symptoms simulated asthma with cough, wheezing, and dyspnea predominating.

6. Pulmonary function test may show airflow obstruction.

7. Methacholine challenge testing was positive.

8. Other types of pulmonary diseases were ruled out.

[a] Clinical criteria for RADS defined by Brooks[18] with minor modification as noted.
[b] Exposure to high-level irritant exposure on one or more occasions not confined to a single workplace event.[33]
[c] Others have used symptom onset up to 7 days after exposure.[34]

---

following longer and less intense irritant exposures. In a group of 71 subjects considered to be at moderate to high risk for RADS after repeated exposures to chlorine at a pulp and paper mill, 82% had persisting respiratory symptoms, 22% had evidence of reduced FEV1, and 41% had nonspecific airways hyperresponsiveness based on methacholine challenge that persisted 18 to 24 months after the end of exposure without clear host predisposition.[40] In contrast, long-term decline in lung function was seen in a longitudinal study of workers exposed to "puffs" of chlorine at a metal production plant; these exposures caused mild symptoms in those with a smoking history of 20-pack-years or more.[41] Kipen and colleagues[21] described a series of 10 cases of adult-onset asthma following "low-dose" irritant exposures, as shown in **Table 2**. Four of the cases were reported due to exposure to acid mist, whereas 4 or 5 of the other irritant exposures potentially also could have been sensitizers. In this series, another 5 cases had been excluded because of a history of asthma before the exposure, although 41% of the cases did meet the investigators' criteria for history of atopy (case history reviewed for seasonal allergy, rhinitis, atopic skin disease, or positive immediate hypersensitivity skin results). Host predisposition was also suggested as a mechanism in the subgroup with "not so sudden" irritant-asthma reported by Brooks and colleagues,[22] in which 88% were atopic (defined as allergen skin testing or radioallergosorbent tests positive, personal history of allergic disease, elevated total immunoglobulin E level, or family history of allergy) and 40% had a history of childhood asthma or asthma that had been quiescent at least 1 year.

It is important to recognize that a single, high-level exposure to a sensitizing chemical with irritant properties may also cause irritant asthma, although it may be difficult to exclude concurrent sensitization when that exposure is not confined to a single event.[18,33] Distinguishing between an immunologic and irritant mechanism can be difficult in the individual patient. This has been handled in a number of different ways: excluding those with exposure to irritants that were also sensitizers,[39,42] analyzing the chemical composition to exclude the presence of sensitizers to determine irritant mechanism,[43] using a specific inhalational challenge (SIC) in the laboratory or workplace to distinguish the two,[44] or including all high-level exposures regardless of SIC

Table 2
Reported low-dose irritant exposures, associated work-exacerbated asthma, and low-dose RADS, along with pH, potential for thermal injury, and sensitizer potential

Author	Outcome	Reported Chemical	High or Low pH	Potential for Thermal Injury	Potential Sensitizer
Chiry et al,[46] 2007	WEA with negative SIC	Flour			+
		Latex			+
		Isocyanates (3)			+
		Glutaraldehyde			+
		Triethanolamine			+
Lemiere et al,[47] 2012	WEA with negative SIC	Ammonia	+		
		Engine exhaust fumes			
		Pyrolysis fumes		?	?
		Metal fumes			?
		Silica			
		Mineral fibers			
		Metal compounds			?
		Animal-derived aerosol			?
		Wood			?
		Flour			+
		Acrylates			+
		Paints, including industrial and motor vehicle			+
		Adhesives			?
		Degreasing stripping agents			
		Hardeners			+
		Isocyanates			+
		Solvents			
Kipen et al,[21] 1994	Low-dose RADS	Bisulfite+SO2			
		Chemistry teaching laboratory	?		?
		Acid mist (4)	+		
		Cutting oil			?
		Cleaning agents			?
		Perfume agents			?
		New carpet installation			?

The "+" refers to the listed chemical exposures that have one or more of the other properties: high or low pH, potential for thermal injury and/or are potential sensitizers. The "?" refers to those chemical exposures that might have one of those properties, but there is insufficient information about the exposure to determine.

Abbreviations: RADS, reactive airways dysfunction syndrome; SIC, specific inhalation challenge; WEA, work-exacerbated asthma.

results.[45] The latter is not inconsistent with the original criteria proposed by Brooks and colleagues.[18] As shown in **Table 1**, many of the irritant exposures reported to cause acute irritant induced asthma are also potential sensitizers. Perhaps more important than establishing mechanism, establishing whether or not there is concurrent immunologic asthma has important implications for the degree of exposure control required for the worker to successfully remain in the workplace.

As described for high-level irritant exposures, lower-level exposures to sensitizing chemicals with irritant properties can also cause asthma either by an irritant or a sensitizing mechanism. Immunologic asthma has been differentiated from irritant-induced asthma in some studies by results from SIC.[46,47] As shown in **Table 2**, many of these irritant exposures in which sensitizers were not automatically excluded are very similar to the exposures reported with acute irritant asthma listed in **Table 1**. In a study by Kogevinas and colleagues,[48] occupations associated with excess risk of occupational asthma included farmers, painters, plastics workers, cleaners, spray painters, and agricultural workers; these are occupations in which there may be concurrent exposures to sensitizers. Overrepresentation of respiratory symptoms and asthma has been reported in workers repeatedly exposed to moderate to low-level irritant exposures that can also be sensitizers, such as cleaning workers[49–51] and hair dressers.[52]

CLINICAL VIGNETTE 3

Sandra Dalton is a 26-year-old woman with a prior history of childhood asthma and seasonal allergic rhinitis. Her asthma improved when she was an adolescent, and she used a bronchodilator only before exercise or for chest symptoms associated with an upper respiratory infection (URI). Six months ago she began a job with a company producing experimental semiconductors. She was responsible for loading panels of chips into a holder; this holder was then lowered into a nitric acid bath before the chips were removed and sent down the assembly line. Her job also involved refilling the nitric acid reservoir when levels were low. Although the bath was covered, it was opened to load and remove the computer chips. The room had an unpleasant acrid odor, and after about 3 months at work, she began to develop more frequent episodes of chest tightness that no longer completely resolved after using her bronchodilator. A recent URI triggered profound cough and wheezing, requiring a burst of oral steroids and the addition of a steroid inhaler to control symptoms. Is the patient's asthma exacerbation work related?

WORK-EXACERBATED ASTHMA

Yes, it is now widely accepted that low-level irritant exposures can exacerbate preexisting asthma.[14–16,24,25] WEA was recently defined by the American Thoracic Society as "preexisting or concurrent asthma that is worsened by workplace conditions," wherein the asthma either predates the exposure (preexisting) or is determined to have occurred independently, but concurrently with the workplace exposure (concurrent).[25] The diagnosis of WEA requires establishment of temporal association between asthma exacerbations and work in a workplace where conditions exist that can exacerbate asthma. WEA is common, reportedly occurring in 23% of adults within a health maintenance organization.[53]

Temporary Exacerbation Versus Permanent Aggravation of Preexisting or Concurrent Asthma

There is an assortment of irritant workplace exposures that may temporarily increase symptoms due to underlying asthma, or indeed any other chronic lung disease. Such increases in symptoms are often mild, temporary, and respond well to simple measures to decrease or avoid exposure, with the occasional additional use of short-acting bronchodilators. Patients with severe underlying asthma may not be tolerant of low level irritants that are present in many different environments. The problem occurs when there are specific exacerbating conditions that exist in the workplace, but the worker does not have control over mitigating them; such workers are often unable to remain in the workplace. A letter to the editor described the long-term impact of WEA in 10 cases 1 to 4 years after a diagnosis of WEA. None had been able to remain in the workplace because of their respiratory symptoms, and they also were unable to obtain any financial compensation from the Quebec Worker Compensation Board.[54] Although it is possible that medical treatment or enhanced ventilation or respiratory protection might have allowed these workers to remain in their jobs, outside of the workers' compensation system, such patients often do not have the authority to effect meaningful decreases in respiratory exposures in the workplace.

As a result, loss of employment, a need to change jobs, and other adverse socioeconomic effects,[55–58] as well as increased use of health care resources and decreased quality of life,[59] have been documented by a growing number of studies of workers after a diagnosis of WEA. If the worker does not return to baseline status despite optimized medical therapy, and reasonable exposure control measures have been implemented, such worsening would be considered a permanent aggravation, rather than a temporary exacerbation.

Although there are considerable data on disability and adverse socioeconomic outcomes in WEA, there are few clinical outcome studies.[25] There are also no clinical outcome data on workers who receive optimized medication therapy and reasonable workplace exposure controls, and their long-term ability to remain within the workplace (ie, the extent to which such cases of WEA could be limited to temporary exacerbations that are not associated with job loss and other socioeconomic disadvantages).

More concrete consideration of permanent aggravation can be made in the context of an acute irritant injury in a worker with preexisting asthma. The original clinical criteria proposed by Brooks and colleagues[18] excluded persons with preceding history of respiratory complaints. In most cases, it is impossible to verify a preexisting lack of airways hyperresponsiveness or airflow limitation. Multiple cases of high-level irritant exposures resulted in asthma that otherwise met the definition of RADS except for a prior history of mild asthma.[22,36,60,61] There is nothing about underlying asthma that would be expected to confer immunity from airways injury following such irritant exposures that cause RADS in a worker with normal airways. Indeed, one might postulate that those with preexisting asthma are even more susceptible to airways injury and persistent effects from irritant exposures, as is suggested by the 76% of subjects with a preexisting history of asthma who had accepted claims for asthma by the Ontario Workers' Compensation Board following high-level irritant exposures.[45] In many cases, with treatment, workers with preexisting asthma will be able to return to their baseline status in the same way as those with no prior history of asthma. In others, the condition does not return to baseline, and there is objective evidence of permanent worsening, such as a change in FEV1, methacholine PC-20, medication requirements, and/or the need for permanent removal from exposure even after optimized medical treatment and implementation of exposure controls. In this setting, the term "acute irritant-aggravated asthma" could be considered to describe the permanent change from the patient's baseline condition.

CHALLENGES IN THE DIAGNOSIS OF IRRITANT-INDUCED VERSUS IRRITANT-AGGRAVATED ASTHMA FROM AN OCCUPATIONAL AND ENVIRONMENTAL MEDICINE PERSPECTIVE DISTINGUISHING WORKERS WITH PREEXISTING OR CONCURRENT ASTHMA FROM NEW-ONSET ASTHMA

There can be difficulty distinguishing between new-onset occupational asthma caused by work, and WEA. For example, in a group of 53 workers with documented reversible airflow limitation or airways hyperresponsiveness and WEA, defined by worsening asthma symptoms at work and a negative SIC, only 20% reported a history of asthma before the exposure.[47] The investigators concluded that although it is often not possible to confirm by objective testing, a proportion of these subjects may suffer not from WEA, but from "low-dose irritant asthma" (ie, new-onset asthma). In another study, clinicians were not able to reliably differentiate the peak flow measurement pattern in workers with new-onset occupational asthma versus WEA on visual inspection or computer analysis.[46] In fact, the US National Institute for Occupational Safety and Health (NIOSH) Sentinel Event Notification Systems for Occupational Risks (SENSOR) program for surveillance of work-related asthma considered new-onset work-related asthma symptoms to be work-initiated asthma, even in the context of preexisting asthma that had been untreated or asymptomatic for at least 2 years before entering the workplace.[62]

Preexisting asymptomatic airways hyperresponsiveness (AHR) is well described as one of the factors that can predispose to asthma, and some investigators have argued that the existence of preexisting AHR precludes a diagnosis of RADS as new-onset asthma. The prevalence of asymptomatic airways hyperresponsiveness has ranged from 4% to 35% of the population depending on the definition used.[63] It is described with[64] and without[65] correlation with eosinophilia, which along with atopy can also predispose to asthma. A prior history of asthma, including childhood asthma, is also defined as preexisting asthma. The extent to which these are preexisting conditions, or simply markers of host risk factors for asthma, remains to be determined.[66]

In many of the US workers' compensation systems, work-related conditions are defined on a medically probable (greater than 50% likely) basis that the need for treatment in a case is the result of a work-related exposure when certain factors are present. These factors include: (1) the work exposure causes a new condition; or (2) the work exposure causes the activation of a previously asymptomatic or latent medical condition to become symptomatic and now require treatment; or (3) the work exposure aggravates a preexisting symptomatic condition that now requires treatment that was not needed before. A helpful approach to determining whether a condition is work-related is recommended by the Colorado Division of Workers' Compensation: would the patient need the recommended treatment if the work exposure had not taken place? If the answer is "no," then the condition is most likely work related.[67] To establish that the worker had preexisting or concurrent asthma, the physician would need to verify an asymptomatic or well-controlled stable asthma pattern that had clearly changed due to a well-defined workplace irritant exposure. It is also incumbent on the physician to rule out the contribution of nonoccupational causes to the asthma exacerbation, such as GERD, infection, or rhinosinusitis.

Defining High-Level Exposure

What constitutes a high-level exposure may or may not be obvious. In cases of very high-level accidental releases where no respiratory protection had been worn, the high-level exposure is obvious. A good example is the massive exposure to airborne alkaline particulates following the World Trade Center collapse in 2001; this led to the development of asthma in many of the first responders.[68–70] When explored, a dose-response has been noted,[28] but in most cases, no industrial hygiene monitoring data or dose reconstruction by an industrial hygienist are available. In less obvious cases, the physician can try to estimate the "dose" that was delivered to the lungs of the individual worker based on the intensity of the irritant exposure, the frequency, and the duration.

Intensity

Intensity is determined by the airborne concentration of the vapor, dust, gas, or fume, as well as the innate irritating properties of the chemical(s). Some chemicals are inherently more irritating than others.[9] For example, those with very low, or worse, very high pH, are extremely irritating. When heated chemicals are inhaled, thermal injury may compound the damage.

A release may or may not be large. A worker very close to the source of a release may have a high concentration in his or her breathing zone that is not shared by others a little farther away, as the concentration of irritants can be fairly quickly dissipated through dilution with ambient air currents. Airborne concentrations will be much higher within a confined space because there is no such potential for dilution. Chemicals with very low vapor pressure can quickly volatilize in considerable quantity, particularly when heated. The size of the chemical particle and its water solubility will determine deposition within the respiratory tract, with the smallest and most water-insoluble chemicals having the greatest potential to reach the lower airways.

However, there does not need to be a release or other recognized event to signal exposure to high-level irritants. Not all workplaces will have appropriate engineering controls in place, such as enclosures and local exhaust ventilation, which can greatly minimize exposure to vapors, dust, gas, and fumes. Such controls need to have been installed and used correctly to be effective. Unrecognized failures of these control measures may result in unrecognized excess exposures, although such exposures may be limited to only a few individuals who work directly in the area. Air monitoring by an industrial hygienist can determine actual airborne concentrations, although if interim control measures have been implemented, these may not reflect the actual concentration at the time of the release or engineering control failure.

The amount of the vapor, dust, gas, or fume that reaches the lungs of the worker will be considerably decreased if respiratory protection is used, but only if it was used and worn correctly, and the exposure did not exceed the respirator's protective limits. A filtering respirator needs to have the correct cartridges for the exposure. For example, particulate filtering cartridges are highly effective in trapping airborne particulates but do not filter out irritant gases. Combined particulate (P100) and organic vapor cartridges are highly effective protection against many gases and vapors, as well as fumes and particulates. Filtering facepiece respirators are considered protective at concentrations up to 10 times the Occupational Safety and Health Administration (OSHA) Permissible Exposure Limit (PEL) for half-face respirators and up to 50 times the PEL with full-face respirators. However, the respirator will only have been effective to that level if it was worn properly sealed to the skin without facial hair, and the adequacy of the seal was confirmed by fit testing.

Frequency

The frequency of the exposure is relevant in considering exposures not confined to a single event, and should be considered along with duration.

Duration

The duration of the exposure before moving to fresh air is another important factor in determining "dose" in both high-level and lower-level exposures. Moderate to heavy physical exertion will increase tidal volume and respiratory rate, thus effectively increasing the amount of the irritant delivered to the lungs per unit of time.

SUMMARY

Acute high-level irritant exposures can cause asthma and exacerbate underlying asthma. Lower-level irritant exposures can at least exacerbate underlying asthma, although there is emerging consensus that recurrent lower-level exposures may also cause asthma. There is overlap between the exposures that have caused acute irritant-induced asthma and WEA, many of which are also sensitizers. What constitutes an excessive level enough to cause asthma from acute high-level or recurrent lower-level accidental releases is not currently defined. New-onset asthma in workers following lower-level irritant exposures, with no prior history of respiratory symptoms or asthma, may well be limited to a subset of "susceptible" hosts, such as those with asymptomatic airways hyperresponsiveness, atopy, and those who "outgrew" childhood asthma. But it is reasonable to consider asthma to more likely than not have been caused by such irritant exposures when previously asymptomatic workers develop symptomatic asthma following clearly defined workplace irritant exposures, the asthma is confirmed by objective testing, and other lung diseases and nonoccupational causes of the asthma have been excluded. This attribution of work-relatedness should also apply to workers with prior well-controlled stable asthma who sustain objectively documented changes in the pattern of their asthma.

Workers with irritant-induced and WEA should receive optimized asthma therapy. Equally important is the reduction and control of their exacerbating workplace exposures. Without the ability to receive this combination treatment, it is likely these cases of WEA will not be limited to temporary exacerbations, but will continue to experience the long-term disability and socioeconomic disadvantage that has been repeatedly observed. The ATS statement on WEA has identified research needs to better define risk factors, biologic mechanisms, and outcomes in WEA,[25] which should help to facilitate necessary interventions in the medical system, as well as to formulate and apply strategies for prevention.

The informed clinician should be prepared to identify and treat both new-onset and work-exacerbated asthma, and to partner with occupational and environmental medicine clinicians to address the challenges inherent in the diagnosis and treatment of irritant-induced and irritant-aggravated asthma.

REFERENCES

1. National Center for Health Statistics. Asthma prevalence, health care use, and mortality: United States, 2003-05. Department of Health and Human Services; 2007.
2. Toren K, Blanc PD. Asthma caused by occupational exposures is common—a systematic analysis of estimates of the population-attributable fraction. BMC Pulm Med 2009;9:7.
3. Vandenplas O, Malo JL, Saetta M, et al. Occupational asthma and extrinsic alveolitis due to isocyanates: current status and perspectives. Br J Ind Med 1993;50: 213–28.
4. Baur X. Hypersensitivity pneumonitis (extrinsic allergic alveolitis) induced by isocyanates. J Allergy Clin Immunol 1995;95:1004–10.
5. Raulf-Heimsoth M, Baur X. Pathomechanisms and pathophysiology of isocyanate-induced diseases—summary of present knowledge. Am J Ind Med 1998;34:137–43.
6. Piirila P, Keskinen H, Anttila S, et al. Allergic alveolitis following exposure to epoxy polyester powder paint containing low amounts (<1%) of acid anhydrides. Eur Respir J 1997;10:948–51.

7. Konichezky S, Schattner A, Ezri T, et al. Thionyl-chloride-induced lung injury and bronchiolitis obliterans. Chest 1993;104:971–3.
8. Markopoulou KD, Cool CD, Elliot TL, et al. Obliterative bronchiolitis: varying presentations and clinicopathological correlation. Eur Respir J 2002;19:20–30.
9. Blanc P, Liu D, Juarez C, et al. Cough in hot pepper workers. Chest 1991;99: 27–32.
10. Ekstrand Y, Ternesten-Hasseus E, Arvidsson M, et al. Sensitivity to environmental irritants and capsaicin cough reaction in patients with a positive methacholine provocation test before and after treatment with inhaled corticosteroids. J Asthma 2011;48:482–9.
11. Schiffman SS, Williams CM. Science of odor as a potential health issue. J Environ Qual 2005;34:129–38.
12. Tarlo SM, Malo JL. An official ATS proceedings: asthma in the workplace: the Third Jack Pepys Workshop on Asthma in the Workplace: answered and unanswered questions. Proc Am Thorac Soc 2009;6:339–49.
13. Vandenplas O, Toren K, Blanc PD. Health and socioeconomic impact of work-related asthma. Eur Respir J 2003;22:689–97.
14. Bernstein IL, Bernstein DI, Chan-Yeung M, et al. Definition and classification of asthma in the workplace. In: Bernstein IL, Chan-Yeung M, Malo JL, et al, editors. Asthma in the workplace. 3rd edition. New York; 2006. p. 1–8.
15. Tarlo SM, Balmes J, Balkissoon R, et al. Diagnosis and management of work-related asthma: American College of Chest Physicians Consensus Statement. Chest 2008;134:1S–41S.
16. Malo JL, Vandenplas O. Definitions and classification of work-related asthma. Immunol Allergy Clin North Am 2011;31:645–62, v.
17. Brooks SM, Lockey J. Reactive airways disease syndrome (RADS): a newly defined occupational disease. Am Rev Respir Dis 1981;123(Suppl):133.
18. Brooks SM, Weiss MA, Bernstein IL. Reactive airways dysfunction syndrome (RADS). Persistent asthma syndrome after high-level irritant exposures. Chest 1985;88:376–84.
19. Alberts WM, do Pico GA. Reactive airways dysfunction syndrome. Chest 1996; 109:1618–26.
20. Francis HC, Prys-Picard CO, Fishwick D, et al. Defining and investigating occupational asthma: a consensus approach. Occup Environ Med 2007;64:361–5.
21. Kipen HM, Blume R, Hutt D. Asthma experience in an occupational and environmental medicine clinic. Low-dose reactive airways dysfunction syndrome. J Occup Med 1994;36:1133–7.
22. Brooks SM, Hammad Y, Richards I, et al. The spectrum of irritant-induced asthma: sudden and not-so-sudden onset and the role of allergy. Chest 1998;113:42–9.
23. Tarlo SM. Workplace irritant exposures: do they produce true occupational asthma? Ann Allergy Asthma Immunol 2003;90:19–23.
24. Goe SK, Henneberger PK, Reilly MJ, et al. A descriptive study of work aggravated asthma. Occup Environ Med 2004;61:512–7.
25. Henneberger PK, Redlich CA, Callahan DB, et al. An official American Thoracic Society statement: work-exacerbated asthma. Am J Respir Crit Care Med 2011;184:368–78.
26. Kern DG, Sherman CB. What is this thing called RADS? Chest 1994;106:1643–4.
27. Kennedy SM. Acquired airway hyperresponsiveness from nonimmunogenic irritant exposure. Occup Med 1992;7:287–300.
28. Kern DG. Outbreak of the reactive airways dysfunction syndrome after a spill of glacial acetic acid. Am Rev Respir Dis 1991;144:1058–64.

29. Malo JL, Cartier A, Boulet LP, et al. Bronchial hyperresponsiveness can improve while spirometry plateaus two to three years after repeated exposure to chlorine causing respiratory symptoms. Am J Respir Crit Care Med 1994;150:1142–5.

30. Chan-Yeung M, Lam S, Kennedy SM, et al. Persistent asthma after repeated exposure to high concentrations of gases in pulpmills. Am J Respir Crit Care Med 1994;149:1676–80.

31. Harkonen H, Nordman H, Korhonen O, et al. Long-term effects of exposure to sulfur dioxide. Lung function four years after a pyrite dust explosion. Am Rev Respir Dis 1983;128:890–3.

32. Piirila PL, Nordman H, Korhonen OS, et al. A thirteen-year follow-up of respiratory effects of acute exposure to sulfur dioxide. Scand J Work Environ Health 1996;22: 191–6.

33. Tarlo SM, Broder I. Irritant-induced occupational asthma. Chest 1989;96:297–300.

34. Cone JE, Wugofski L, Balmes JR, et al. Persistent respiratory health effects after a metam sodium pesticide spill. Chest 1994;106:500–8.

35. Takeda N, Maghni K, Daigle S, et al. Long-term pathologic consequences of acute irritant-induced asthma. J Allergy Clin Immunol 2009;124:975–981.e1.

36. Demeter SL, Cordasco EM, Guidotti TL. Permanent respiratory impairment and upper airway symptoms despite clinical improvement in patients with reactive airways dysfunction syndrome. Sci Total Environ 2001;270:49–55.

37. Malo J, L'Archeveque L, Gastellanos L, et al. Long-term outcomes of acute irritant-induced asthma. Am J Respir Crit Care Med 2009;179:923–8.

38. Maghni K, Lemiere C, Ghezzo H. Airway inflammation after cessation of exposure to agents causing occupational asthma. Am J Respir Crit Care Med 2004;169: 367–72.

39. Brooks S, Hammad Y, Richards I, et al. The Spectrum of irritant-induced asthma. Chest 1998;113:42–9.

40. Bherer L, Cushman R, Courteau JP, et al. Survey of construction workers repeatedly exposed to chlorine over a three to six month period in a pulpmill: II. Follow up of affected workers by questionnaire, spirometry, and assessment of bronchial responsiveness 18 to 24 months after exposure ended. Occup Environ Med 1994;51:225–8.

41. Gautrin D, Leroyer C, Infante-Rivard C, et al. Longitudinal assessment of airway caliber and responsiveness in workers exposed to chlorine. Am J Respir Crit Care Med 1999;160:1232–7.

42. Wheeler S, Rosenstock L, Barnhart S. A case series of 71 patients referred to a hospital-based occupational and environmental medicine clinic for occupational asthma. West J Med 1998;168:98–104.

43. Burge PS, Moore VC, Robertson AS. Sensitization and irritant-induced occupational asthma with latency are clinically indistinguishable. Occup Med 2012;62: 129–33.

44. Leroyer C, Dewitte JD, Bassanets A, et al. Occupational asthma due to chromium. Respiration 1998;65:403–5.

45. Chatkin JM, Tarlo SM, Liss G, et al. The outcome of asthma related to workplace irritant exposures: a comparison of irritant-induced asthma and irritant aggravation of asthma. Chest 1999;116:1780–5.

46. Chiry S, Cartier A, Malo JL, et al. Comparison of peak expiratory flow variability between workers with work-exacerbated asthma and occupational asthma. Chest 2007;132:483–8.

47. Lemiere C, Begin D, Camus M, et al. Occupational risk factors associated with work-exacerbated asthma in Quebec. Occup Environ Med 2012;00:1–7.

48. Kogevinas M, Anto JM, Sunyer J, et al. Occupational asthma in Europe and other industrialised areas: a population-based study. European Community Respiratory Health Survey Study Group. Lancet 1999;353:1750–4.
49. Quirce S, Barranco P. Cleaning agents and asthma. J Investig Allergol Clin Immunol 2010;20:542–50 [quiz: 2p following 50].
50. Karjalainen A, Martikainen R, Karjalainen J, et al. Excess incidence of asthma among Finnish cleaners employed in different industries. Eur Respir J 2002;19:90–5.
51. Rosenman KD, Reilly MJ, Schill DP, et al. Cleaning products and work-related asthma. J Occup Environ Med 2003;45:556–63.
52. Moscato G, Galdi E. Asthma and hairdressers. Curr Opin Allergy Clin Immunol 2006;6:91–5.
53. Henneberger PK, Derk SJ, Sama SR, et al. The frequency of workplace exacerbation among health maintenance organisation members with asthma. Occup Environ Med 2006;63:551–7.
54. Pelissier S, Chaboillez S, Teolis L, et al. Outcome of subjects diagnosed with occupational asthma and work-aggravated asthma after removal from exposure. J Occup Environ Med 2006;48:656–9.
55. Vandenplas O, Henneberger PK. Socioeconomic outcomes in work-exacerbated asthma. Curr Opin Allergy Clin Immunol 2007;7:236–41.
56. Larbanois A, Jamart J, Delwiche JP, et al. Socioeconomic outcome of subjects experiencing asthma symptoms at work. Eur Respir J 2002;19:1107–13.
57. Cannon J, Cullinan P, Newman TA. Consequences of occupational asthma. BMJ 1995;311:602–3.
58. Blanc PD, Ellbjar S, Janson C, et al. Asthma-related work disability in Sweden. The impact of workplace exposures. Am J Respir Crit Care Med 1999;160: 2028–33.
59. Lemiere C. Occupational and work-exacerbated asthma: similarities and differences. Expert Rev Respir Med 2007;1:43–9.
60. Boulet LP. Increases in airway responsiveness following acute exposure to respiratory irritants. Reactive airway dysfunction syndrome or occupational asthma? Chest 1988;94:476–81.
61. Moore BB, Sherman M. Chronic reactive airway disease following acute chlorine gas exposure in an asymptomatic atopic patient. Chest 1991;100:855–6.
62. Jajosky RA, Harrison R, Reinisch F, et al. Surveillance of work-related asthma in selected U.S. states using surveillance guidelines for state health departments—California, Massachusetts, Michigan, and New Jersey, 1993–1995. MMWR CDC Surveill Summ 1999;48:1–20.
63. Boulet LP. Asymptomatic airway hyperresponsiveness: a curiosity or an opportunity to prevent asthma? Am J Respir Crit Care Med 2003;167:371–8.
64. Schwartz N, Grossman A, Levy Y, et al. Correlation between eosinophil count and methacholine challenge test in asymptomatic subjects. J Asthma 2012;49: 336–41.
65. Boulet LP, Prince P, Turcotte H, et al. Clinical features and airway inflammation in mild asthma versus asymptomatic airway hyperresponsiveness. Respir Med 2006;100:292–9.
66. Laprise C, Laviolette M, Boutet M, et al. Asymptomatic airway hyperresponsiveness: relationships with airway inflammation and remodelling. Eur Respir J 1999; 14:63–73.
67. State of Colorado Department of Labor and Employment Division of Workers' Compensation Level II Accreditation Course and Curriculum. Available at http://www.colorado.gov/cs/Satellite/CDLE-WorkComp/CDLE/1240336932511.

68. Prezant DJ, Levin S, Kelly KJ, et al. Upper and lower respiratory diseases after occupational and environmental disasters. Mt Sinai J Med 2008;75:89–100.
69. Prezant DJ, Weiden M, Banauch GI, et al. Cough and bronchial responsiveness in firefighters at the World Trade Center site. N Engl J Med 2002;347:806–15.
70. Banauch GI, Alleyne D, Sanchez R, et al. Persistent hyperreactivity and reactive airway dysfunction in firefighters at the World Trade Center. Am J Respir Crit Care Med 2003;168:54–62.

COPD Exacerbations
Causes, Prevention, and Treatment

Alex J. Mackay, MBBS, BSc (Hons), MRCP*, John R. Hurst, PhD, FRCP

KEYWORDS

- Chronic obstructive pulmonary disease • Exacerbation • Respiratory viruses
- Bacteria

KEY POINTS

- Respiratory viruses (in particular rhinovirus) and bacteria both play a major role in the etiology of exacerbate COPD.
- A distinct group of patients appears susceptible to frequent exacerbations, irrespective of disease severity and this phenotype is stable over time.
- Many current therapeutic strategies help reduce exacerbation frequency.

Chronic obstructive pulmonary disease (COPD) is associated with episodes of acute deterioration in respiratory health termed "exacerbations." Exacerbations are characterized by a worsening of symptoms from the usual stable state, especially dyspnea, increased sputum volume, and purulence. When diagnosing COPD exacerbations, clinicians must also exclude other causes for respiratory deterioration, such as pneumothoraces, pulmonary emboli, and pneumonia, using clinical examination and appropriate investigations if required. Exacerbations are among the most common causes of emergency medical hospital admission in the United Kingdom[1] (and elsewhere) and the rate at which they occur seems to reflect an independent susceptibility phenotype.[2] Exacerbations are important events in the natural history of COPD that help drive lung function decline,[3,4] increase the risk of cardiovascular events,[5] and are responsible for much of the morbidity[6] and mortality[7] associated with this highly prevalent condition.

FREQUENT EXACERBATOR PHENOTYPE

Patients with a history of frequent exacerbations exhibit faster decline in lung function,[3] have worse quality of life,[6] have increased risk of hospitalization,[8] and have

This article originally appeared in *Med Clin N Am 96:4(2012)*.
Financial Disclosures: Dr Hurst has received support to attend meetings or speaker and advisory fees from AstraZeneca, Bayer, Boehringer Ingelheim, Chiesi, GlaxoSmithKline, and Pfizer.
Academic Unit of Respiratory Medicine, Royal Free Campus, UCL Medical School, Rowland Hill Street, London NW3 2PF, UK
* Corresponding author.
E-mail address: alexander.mackay@ucl.ac.uk

greater mortality (**Fig. 1**).[7] Therefore, it is important to identify patients at risk of frequent exacerbations. Exacerbations become more frequent and severe as COPD severity increases.[9] However, a distinct group of patients seems to be susceptible to exacerbations, irrespective of disease severity, and the major determinant of exacerbation frequency is a history of prior exacerbations.[2] This phenotype of susceptibility to exacerbations is stable over time and is seen across all severity of airflow obstruction,[2] suggesting that patients with the frequent exacerbator phenotype are prone to exacerbations as a result of intrinsic susceptibility, and develop exacerbations when exposed to particular triggers, such as respiratory infections.

Exacerbations are associated with increased systemic and airway inflammation and may be triggered by bacterial and respiratory viral infections. They may also be precipitated by environmental factors (**Fig. 2**).

VIRAL INFECTIONS
Rhinovirus

Rhinovirus is responsible for the common cold and initial evidence that respiratory viral infections were important triggers of COPD exacerbations came from the association of coryzal symptoms with exacerbations. Seemungal and colleagues[10] found that up to 64% of exacerbations were associated with a symptomatic cold occurring up to 18 days before exacerbation onset. Additionally, exacerbations associated with dyspnea and coryza at onset are associated with larger falls in peak flow, prolonged recovery times, and higher levels of airway inflammatory markers (interleukin [IL]-6).[11,12]

Studies using molecular biology polymerase chain reaction techniques have provided further evidence of the role of rhinovirus in the cause of COPD exacerbations. In studies from the London COPD cohort, up to 40% of exacerbations were associated with respiratory viral infections. Rhinovirus was the most common respiratory virus detected and found in 58% of viral exacerbations.[10] Rohde and colleagues[13] corroborated these findings in a separate study of hospitalized patients, detecting respiratory viruses in 56% of exacerbations. Rhinovirus was again the most prevalent virus, being detected in 36% of virus-associated exacerbations.

Experimental Rhinovirus Infection Models

Mallia and colleagues[14] have used experimental rhinovirus infection to provide evidence of a direct causal relationship between respiratory virus infection and acute exacerbations of COPD. In that study, 13 subjects with COPD and 13 control subjects with a similar smoking history but normal lung function were closely observed after

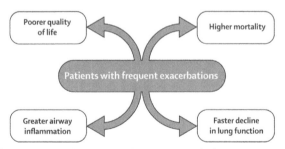

Fig. 1. Effect of COPD exacerbations in the group with frequent exacerbations. (*From* Wedzicha JA, Seemungal TA. COPD exacerbations: defining their cause and prevention. Lancet 2007;370(9589):786–96; with permission.)

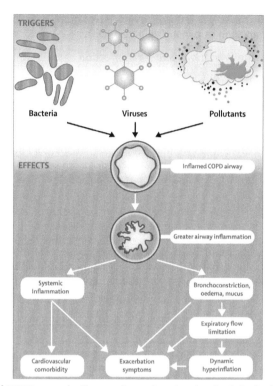

Fig. 2. Triggers of COPD exacerbations and associated pathophysiologic changes leading to increased respiratory symptoms. (*From* Wedzicha JA, Seemungal TA. COPD exacerbations: defining their cause and prevention. Lancet 2007;370(9589):786–96; with permission.)

infection with rhinovirus serotype 16. Daily upper and lower respiratory symptom scores were increased significantly above baseline levels and were significantly greater in the COPD group compared with control subjects. Postbronchodilator peak expiratory flow fell and in blood and airway inflammatory markers increased significantly from baseline in patients with COPD but not control subjects. Nasal lavage virus load was significantly higher in the COPD group compared with control subjects and peak sputum virus load in subjects with COPD correlated positively with peak serum C-reactive protein concentration and sputum inflammatory markers (neutrophils, IL-6, IL-8, neutrophil elastase, and tumor necrosis factor-α). Furthermore, there was a temporal relationship between virus detection in the respiratory tract and the onset of symptoms and airflow obstruction, and virus clearance was followed by clinical recovery. Thus, Mallia and colleagues[14] provide direct evidence that the symptomatic and physiologic changes seen at acute exacerbations of COPD can be precipitated by rhinovirus infection.

Susceptibility to Virus-Induced Exacerbations

Defective immunity may lead to increased susceptibility to virus-induced exacerbations. Interferon-β is an essential component of antirhinoviral immunity and Mallia and colleagues[14] have reported impaired interferon-β response to rhinovirus infection in COPD. Furthermore, cells from patients with COPD manifest increased viral titer and copy numbers after rhinovirus infection compared with control subjects[15] and intercellular adhesion molecule-1, the rhinovirus major group receptor, is up-regulated on the bronchial epithelium of patients with COPD.[16]

Seasonal Environmental Variations and Viral Infection

In the Northern hemisphere, COPD exacerbations are more common in the winter months and may also be more severe, because small but significant falls in lung function in patients with COPD occur with a reduction in outdoor temperature.[17] The increase in exacerbations may be caused by the increasing prevalence of respiratory viruses in low temperature winter months or increased susceptibility to upper respiratory tract virus infections in cold weather. In children, respiratory syncytial virus (RSV) outbreaks cause a significant increase in hospital admissions during the winter season[18] and increased RSV activity has been observed when temperatures decrease.[19]

RSV

Seemungal and colleagues[10] detected RSV in nasal aspirates at exacerbation, although more patients had RSV detected in the stable state than at exacerbation (23.5% vs 14.2%). Stable patients in whom RSV has been detected have elevated inflammatory markers, more severely impaired gas exchange (higher $Paco_2$) and accelerated lung function decline.[10,20] Thus, RSV may also be a cause of chronic airway infection in COPD.

Influenza Virus

Influenza has been detected relatively infrequently at COPD exacerbation,[10] though this may relate to widespread use of influenza immunization for patients with chronic lung disease. In studies of older patients with chronic lung disease, those not vaccinated with influenza had twice the hospitalization rate in the influenza season compared with the noninfluenza season.[21] This highlights the importance of influenza vaccination in patients with COPD and suggests that influenza may still be an important etiologic factor during influenza epidemics.

BACTERIAL INFECTIONS
Species

Bacteria are isolated from sputum using standard culture techniques in 40% to 60% of exacerbations.[22] The three most common species isolated in COPD exacerbations are Haemophilus influenzae, Moraxella catarrhalis, and Streptococcus pneumoniae. Less frequently, exacerbations may be caused by Pseudomonas aeruginosa, gram-negative Enterobacteriacea, Staphylococcus aureus, Haemophilus parainfluenzae, and Haemophilus hemolyticus.[23–25]

Sputum Characteristics

Some of the earliest evidence supporting a causative role for bacteria in COPD exacerbations came from antibiotic studies, including the seminal paper by Anthonisen and colleagues,[26] which identified exacerbation features predictive of benefit from antibiotics. Patients with increased dyspnea, sputum volume, and sputum purulence showed a significant benefit with antibiotic therapy, whereas those with only one of these three features showed none. After this paper, studies related sputum characteristics to the presence of bacteria and bacterial load. Theoretically, airway bacterial infection should be accompanied by an influx of neutrophils, resulting in a change in secretions from mucoid to purulent, because neutrophil-derived myeloperoxidase is green. Antibiotic therapy, by reducing bacterial load, should reverse this process.[27]

In studies during exacerbations of COPD, positive bacterial cultures were obtained from 84% of patients if sputum was purulent at presentation but only 38% if the sputum was mucoid ($P<.0001$). Moreover, the median bacterial load for positive purulent culture samples was significantly higher than for mucoid samples. When the same patients were reexamined in the stable state after antibiotics, sputum color improved significantly in the group who presented with purulent sputum. In purulent exacerbations a clear relationship was demonstrated between semiquantitative neutrophil count and sputum color. The presence of green (purulent) sputum was 94.4% sensitive and 77% specific for a high bacterial load ($>10^7$ colony forming units per milliliter).[27]

Colonization

Darker sputum color in stable COPD may reflect bronchial bacterial colonization,[28] which has traditionally been characterized as the isolation by culture of significant numbers of bacteria in samples obtained from the lower airways of patients with COPD when clinically stable.[29] Bacteria in the lower airways have been hypothesized to disrupt host defense mechanisms leading to a vicious cycle of epithelial cell injury, defective mucociliary clearance, chronic mucous hypersecretion, and inflammatory cell infiltration, further damaging host defenses and leading to bacterial adherence and growth.[23] This mechanism may explain why colonization in the stable state has been associated with increased exacerbation frequency (**Fig. 3**).[30] However, recent technologic advances in bacterial detection have challenged conventional thinking and definitions in the field of bacterial colonization.

Molecular Analysis Techniques

Classically, it was thought the lower airways were sterile in healthy patients; however, the development of culture-independent molecular techniques using 16S-rRNA techniques has challenged this assumption. The 16S-rRNA gene is a section of prokaryotic

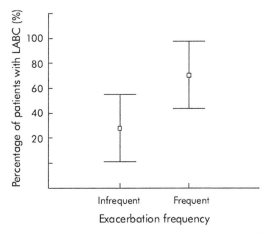

Fig. 3. Relationship between lower airway bacterial colonization (LABC) by a possible pathogen in induced sputum and frequent (>2.58 exacerbations per year; n = 14) and infrequent exacerbations (<2.58 exacerbations per year; n = 14) with 95% confidence intervals. (*From* Patel IS, Seemungal TA, Wilks M, et al. Relationship between bacterial colonisation and the frequency, character, and severity of COPD exacerbations. Thorax 2002;57(9):759–64; with permission.)

DNA found in all bacteria. 16S-rRNA gene sequences contain hypervariable regions that can provide species-specific signature sequences useful for bacterial identification. Consequently, 16S rRNA gene sequencing provides a potentially more accurate alternative to traditional methods of bacterial identification. Hilty and colleagues[31] used molecular analysis of the polymorphic bacterial 16S-rRNA gene to characterize the composition of bacterial communities from the airways of patients with asthma, patients with COPD, and healthy control subjects. Over 5000 16S rRNA bacterial sequences were identified from 43 subjects and the bronchial tree of all patient groups was nonsterile. However, proteobacteria, especially *Haemophilus* sp, were much more frequently identified in the bronchi of patients with asthma and patients with COPD compared with control subjects, suggesting that the bronchial tree contains a characteristic microbial flora that differs between health and disease. Further studies using these techniques have also revealed that there are significant microanatomic differences in bacterial communities within the same lung of subjects with advanced COPD.[32] These techniques are exciting developments in the study of bacteria in patients with COPD, but should be interpreted with caution because studies using these methods have been conducted on small numbers of patients[31,32] and the clinical applicability of the results remains uncertain.

Bacterial Load

The prevalence of potentially pathogenic microorganisms and airway bacterial load in sputum have been shown to increase from stable state to exacerbation. The most frequently isolated organism is *H influenzae*, followed by *M catarrhalis* and *S pneumoniae*.[33] Studies using protected brush specimens collected in the stable state and at exacerbation have also demonstrated an increased prevalence of positive bacterial cultures at exacerbation. In the stable state, patients colonized by potentially pathogenic microorganisms on culture had greater disease severity (reduced mean forced expiratory volume in 1 second [FEV_1]% predicted) and multivariate analyses demonstrated that a high potentially pathogenic microorganism load in lower airway secretions was a major determinant of exacerbation risk and lung function impairment.[34]

Strain Changes

Strain changes may play an important role in the cause of COPD exacerbations. In a prospective study, Sethi and colleagues[25] hypothesized that acquisition of a new bacterial strain would be associated with an exacerbation of COPD and so collected sputum samples from 81 outpatients with moderate to severe COPD on a monthly basis and at exacerbation. Molecular typing of sputum showed that isolation of a new strain of a pathogen (*H influenzae*, *M catarrhalis*, and *S pneumoniae*) was associated with a significant increase in the risk of exacerbation. These findings were proposed as a mechanism to explain recurrent bacterial exacerbations of COPD, the authors speculating that after a first exacerbation, patients develop a protective immune response that is strain specific. Therefore, acquisition of a different strain from the same bacterial species may still lead to a second exacerbation. However, not all exacerbations were associated with strain change, and not all strain changes were associated with exacerbation.

Controversy exists regarding the relative contributions made by exacerbation load and strain change to the cause of COPD exacerbations. Sethi and colleagues[35] further explored this issue by examining sputum from 104 patients when stable and at exacerbation over a period of 81 months. Among preexisting strains, no differences were found between exacerbation and stable bacterial load for *H influenzae*. *M catarrhalis* was present at significantly lower concentrations during exacerbation with a similar trend observed for *S pneumoniae*. However, for *H influenzae* and *M catarrhalis* (but not *S pneumoniae*) increased load of new strains was seen during exacerbation compared with during stable visits. In the case of *H influenzae*, bacterial load increased significantly from $10^{7.28}$ to $10^{7.76}$ colony forming units per milliliter. When the same strain was isolated during stable and exacerbation visits paired analysis also showed a significant increase in load for *H influenzae*. The observed increases of around 0.5 log in magnitude, although representing a small relative change,[35] equate to a 202% or threefold increase in absolute bacterial numbers,[36] suggesting that changes in bacterial load remain an important mechanism for some exacerbations.

Interaction of Bacteria and Viruses

Frequent exacerbators have a higher incidence of lower airway bacterial colonization[30] and bacteria may also play a role in susceptibility to viral infection in COPD. *H influenzae* increases expression of intercellular adhesion molecule-1 and Toll-like receptor-3, and augments binding of rhinovirus to cultured human airway epithelial cells.[37] Therefore, patients colonized with bacteria may be more susceptible to the development of virally triggered exacerbations.

Wilkinson and colleagues[33] demonstrated a synergistic effect of viral and bacterial infections at exacerbation in patients with COPD. Exacerbation symptoms and FEV_1 decline were more severe in the presence of bacteria and colds (as a surrogate of viral infection) than with a cold or bacterial pathogen alone, and exacerbations associated with human rhinovirus and *H influenzae* exhibited a greater bacterial load and inflammation than those without both pathogens. Patients hospitalized because of COPD exacerbations also have more marked lung function impairment and increased length of stay in the context of bacterial and viral coinfection.[38]

ENVIRONMENTAL FACTORS
Air Pollution

Epidemiologic data supports a role for air pollution in the cause of some COPD exacerbations with studies showing an increased risk of hospitalization for COPD with increased levels of pollutants.[39–41] Air pollution likely causes COPD exacerbations through modulation of airway inflammation and immunity. Diesel exhaust induces airway inflammation in healthy volunteers as characterized by an increased percentage of sputum neutrophils, IL-6, and methylhistamine.[42] Furthermore, diesel exhaust reduces T-cell activation and induces migration of alveolar macrophages into the airspaces.[43]

EXACERBATION PREVENTION

There are now a wide range of pharmacologic and nonpharmacologic interventions documented to reduce exacerbation frequency or hospitalization in COPD (**Table 1**). However, there remains a real need for further novel interventions because current approaches are not completely effective, even when targeted and used optimally.

PHARMACOLOGIC THERAPIES

Conceptually, some pharmacotherapy (eg, a vaccine) may be delivered once with lasting effect on reducing exacerbations, whereas other interventions need to be administered continually for that effect to be maintained.

Table 1
Interventions to reduce exacerbation frequency or hospitalization in patients with COPD

Pharmacologic	Nonpharmacologic
Inhaled corticosteroids	Lung volume reduction surgery
Long-acting bronchodilators	Home oxygen
Phosphodiesterase inhibitors	Ventilatory support
Theophyllines	Pulmonary rehabilitation
Long-term antibiotics	
Mucolytics	
Vaccination	

Vaccination

The largest study of the efficacy of influenza vaccination was conducted retrospectively using data pooled from 18 cohort studies of community-dwelling elderly patients over 10 influenza seasons. In this data set composed of 713,872 person-seasons of observation, influenza vaccination was associated with a 27% reduction in the risk of hospitalization for pneumonia or influenza and a 48% reduction in the risk of death.[44] The same authors also conducted a 2-year retrospective cohort study of elderly patients with diagnosis of chronic lung disease to assess the health-economic benefits of pneumococcal vaccination.[45] Pneumococcal vaccination was associated with significantly lower risks of hospitalization for pneumonia and death. However, a randomized controlled trial of pneumococcal polysaccharide vaccine in patients with COPD demonstrated no significant reduction in rates of community-acquired pneumonia when the entire study population was analyzed.[46] Subanalyses of the data showed a reduction in the incidence of community-acquired pneumonia in those patients younger than age 65 years and those with severe airflow obstruction, although no mortality benefit was demonstrated.[46] Data also suggest an additive benefit of combined influenza and pneumococcal vaccination[45] and hence both vaccines are recommended to all patients with COPD.[47] It is important to note that these studies have not specifically addressed exacerbations of COPD.

Bacterial immunostimulation has also been advocated as a method to prevent exacerbations of COPD and reduce the severity and duration of acute episodes. OM-85 BV (Bronchovaxom) is a detoxified immunoactive bacterial extract that has been examined in multiple trials; however, assessment of its efficacy is hampered by heterogeneity of study design and conflicting results.[48–51] Furthermore, it is not known if any protective effects seen are additive to other conventional treatments and thus larger and longer trials are required before this vaccine can be recommended as part of the routine clinical management of COPD.[52]

Inhaled Corticosteroids and Long-Acting Bronchodilators

The Inhaled Steroid in Obstructive Lung Disease in Europe study was performed primarily to assess the effect of inhaled corticosteroids (ICS) on the rate of FEV_1 decline in patients with moderate-to-severe COPD. Although this primary outcome was negative, a 25% reduction in exacerbation frequency was noted in the group who received fluticasone.[53] Long-acting β-agonists (LABA) also reduce exacerbation frequency and in the Toward A Revolution in COPD Health (TORCH) study, in which 6112 patients were followed over 3 years, inhaled fluticasone and salmeterol reduced exacerbation frequency when administered separately compared with placebo.[54]

In the same study, the combination of fluticasone and salmeterol (SFC) reduced exacerbation frequency further still, in addition to improving health status and lung function compared with placebo. The annual rate of moderate and severe exacerbations in the placebo group was 1.13 per year, compared with 0.97 for salmeterol, 0.93 for fluticasone, and 0.85 in patients receiving SFC. The combination of ICS and LABA also resulted in fewer hospital admissions over the study period and trended toward a mortality benefit. Reduction in exacerbation frequency has been found for other ICS, and other LABA, singly and in combination. New drugs in development include once-daily ICS and LABA.

Long-acting antimuscarinics (LAMA) also reduce exacerbation frequency. In the Understanding Potential Long-Term Impacts on Function with Tiotropium trial 5993 patients were randomized to tiotropium or placebo over 4 years, with concomitant therapy allowed. Although the primary end point of the trial (a reduction in rate of decline in FEV_1) was negative, the group of patients randomized to tiotropium in addition to usual care had a significant reduction in exacerbation frequency, related hospitalizations, and respiratory failure.[55] Because this trial involved the addition of tiotropium to existing therapy, which could include combination preparations of ICS and LABA, many patients were in effect on triple combination of therapy.

Triple combination therapy is commonly prescribed in advanced COPD. This approach was examined in the OPTIMAL study, which examined whether combining tiotropium with salmeterol or SFC improved outcomes compared with tiotropium alone in patients with moderate to severe COPD.[56] The primary outcome was negative, because the addition of SFC to tiotropium therapy did not statistically influence rates of COPD exacerbation. However, triple combination therapy did improve lung function, quality of life, and hospitalization rates compared with tiotropium plus placebo. In keeping with the TORCH study, drop-outs in the placebo arm may have affected the study: more than 40% of patients who received tiotropium plus placebo and tiotropium plus salmeterol discontinued therapy prematurely, and many crossed over to treatment with open-label inhaled steroids or LABA.

An important clinical question is which combination of therapies is most effective for different patients. Network analysis techniques have assessed the relative effectiveness of competing inhaled drug regimens for the prevention of COPD exacerbations.[57] Based on 35 trials, all inhaled drug regimens (LABA, LAMA, and ICS, alone and in combination) significantly reduced exacerbations but there were no significant differences between them. In subanalyses, in patients with FEV_1 less than or equal to 40% predicted, LAMA, ICS, and combination treatment reduced exacerbations significantly compared with LABA alone, but not if FEV_1 was greater than 40% predicted. This effect modification was significant for ICS and combination treatment but not for LAMA suggesting that combination treatment may be more effective than LABA alone in patients with a low FEV_1.

Phosphodiesterase Inhibitors

There is some evidence that theophyllines reduce exacerbation frequency.[58,59] However, they are nonselective phosphodiesterase inhibitors, potentially toxic with the need to monitor plasma levels, and with potential for interaction with other medication, restricting therapeutic use. This is a particularly important consideration in elderly patients because of differences in pharmacokinetics, increased prevalence of comorbidities, and concomitant medications. Therefore, theophyllines should only be used after a trial of other more effective therapies (LABA, LAMA, or ICS), or in patients unable to use inhaled therapy. If prescribed, the theophylline dose must be monitored or reduced at exacerbation when macrolide or fluoroquinolones antibiotics are used.[47]

Selective phosphodiesterase-4 inhibitors inhibit the airway inflammatory processes associated with COPD and have a considerably better side effect profile than theophylline. Evidence from a pooled analysis of two large placebo-controlled, double-blind multicentre trials revealed a significant reduction of 17% in the frequency of moderate (glucocorticoid treated) or severe (hospitalization or death) exacerbations.[60] However, the study design of these trials limits the generalizability: patients had to have an FEV_1 less than 50% (Global Initiative for Chronic Obstructive Lung Disease stages 3 and 4); bronchitic symptoms; and a history of exacerbations. Furthermore, only LABA were allowed as maintenance therapy during the study and there are currently no comparator studies of roflumilast with ICS. Discontinuations because of adverse events were more common in the roflumilast group than in the placebo group, the most frequent adverse events leading to discontinuation (with the exception of COPD) being diarrhea, nausea, and headache. Weight loss was also noted in the roflumilast group, with a mean reduction of 2.1 kg after 1 year, which was greatest in obese patients. Concerns regarding tolerability and side effects of roflumilast therapy may have limited its clinical use.

Long-Term Antibiotics

At present there is insufficient evidence to recommend routine prophylactic antibiotic therapy in the management of stable COPD. However, recent studies have shown promise, particularly those involving macrolides, which have anti-inflammatory and antimicrobial properties. Erythromycin reduced the frequency of moderate or severe exacerbations (treated with systemic steroids or antibiotics, or hospitalized) and shortened exacerbation length when taken twice daily over 12 months by patients with moderate-to-severe COPD.[61] The macrolide azithromycin has been used as prophylaxis in patients with cystic fibrosis and is also suitable for use in patients with COPD for exacerbation prevention. A large United States trial of more than 1500 patients with COPD at high risk of exacerbations recently reported that when added to usual treatment, azithromycin taken daily for 1 year decreased the frequency of exacerbations and improved quality of life. However, patients in the azithromycin intervention group were more likely to become colonized with macrolide-resistant organisms and suffer hearing decrements.[62] Ongoing concerns regarding the development of antibiotic resistance have led to trials of alternative, pulsed antibiotic regimens. Intermittent pulsed moxifloxacin when given to stable patients significantly reduced exacerbation frequency in a per-protocol population, and in a post hoc subgroup of patients with bronchitis at baseline. However, this reduction did not meet statistical significance in the intention-to-treat analysis and further work is required in this area.[63]

Mucolytics

The routine use of these agents is not currently recommended. Some evidence exists that mucolytics, such as carbocysteine, may reduce exacerbation frequency in selected patients with viscous sputum.[64] However, it is not certain if these treatments provide additional benefit to patients already being treated with LABA or ICS.

Novel Anti-Inflammatory Drugs

COPD is an inflammatory condition associated with relative steroid resistance and approaches to restore steroid sensitivity may lead to novel future therapies.[65] Histone deacetylase-2 is reduced in airway tissue from patients with COPD compared with healthy nonsmokers and has been implicated in impaired sensitivity to corticosteroids.[66]

Increasing histone deacetylase-2 expression or activation may be a potential avenue to reversing corticosteroid subsensitivity in COPD. Low doses of oral theophylline have been shown to increase histone deacetylase-2 expression in alveolar macrophages from patients with COPD[67,68] and so potentially may restore corticosteroid responsiveness in vivo.

There is evidence of significantly increased phosphoinositide-3-kinase activity in peripheral blood monocytes from patients with COPD compared with smokers and normal control subjects, a pathway that is also associated with reduced corticosteroid sensitivity.[69] The addition of a phosphoinositide-3-kinase inhibitor has been shown to restore steroid sensitivity toward normal[70] and a number of phosphoinositide-3-kinase–delta inhibitors are currently under development.

Alveolar macrophages from patients with COPD demonstrate increased p38 mitogen-activated protein kinase activity.[71] In patients with COPD, selective p38 (p38 mitogen-activated protein kinase) inhibitors reduce lipopolysaccharide-induced cytokine production in alveolar macrophages and synergistically increase the cytokine suppressive effects of dexamethasone.[72]

NONPHARMACOLOGIC THERAPIES
Lung Volume Reduction Surgery

The National Emphysema Treatment Trial reported that lung volume reduction surgery can improve morbidity and mortality in a subset of patients with COPD who have predominantly upper-lobe emphysema and low baseline exercise capacity.[73] A retrospective investigation of data from the same study also showed that lung volume reduction surgery reduces the frequency of COPD exacerbations, possibly through postoperative improvement in lung function[74] and reduction in dynamic hyperinflation. Therefore, this therapeutic option should be explored in selected eligible patients.

Home Oxygen and Ventilatory Support

Although a specific effect of oxygen on reducing exacerbations has not been demonstrated, long-term oxygen therapy has a proved mortality benefit in COPD.[75,76] Furthermore, under-prescription of long-term oxygen therapy where indicated was associated with increased hospital admissions.[77] Domiciliary noninvasive ventilation (NIV) may also improve survival for patients with COPD with hypercapneic respiratory failure[78]; however, controlled trials in this area with regard to exacerbations are also lacking.

Pulmonary Rehabilitation

There is evidence that multiprofessional exercise and education pulmonary rehabilitation programs reduce hospitalization rates in COPD, while improving health status and functional capacity.[79] Maintenance programs may be necessary to maintain these benefits.

Exacerbation therapy is administered in a step-wise model as previously mentioned (**Fig. 4**).[80] The mainstay of exacerbation therapy is an increase in the dose and frequency of short-acting bronchodilators and systemic corticosteroids. Antibiotics are reserved for exacerbations associated with increasing sputum volume or purulence.

Self Management

Patient education is vital to improved management of COPD exacerbations. Rapid recognition of exacerbation symptoms and earlier treatment improves recovery and reduces the risk of hospitalization.[81] These findings have been incorporated into

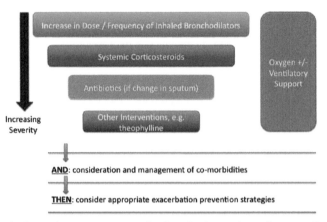

Fig. 4. General scheme for management of a chronic obstructive pulmonary disease (COPD) exacerbation. (*From* Hurst JR, Wedzicha JA. Management and prevention of chronic obstructive pulmonary disease exacerbations: a state of the art review. BMC Med 2009;7:40.)

many patient self-management plans and programs that are designed to enable patients to respond appropriately to the first signs of an exacerbation without leading to overtreatment of minor symptom variations. Patients at high risk of exacerbations can be provided with a course of "rescue" antibiotics and corticosteroids to keep at home for use as part of a self-management strategy and instructed to commence oral corticosteroid therapy if their increased dyspnea interferes with activities of daily living, either independently or after seeking advice from a healthcare professional. Antibiotics should be started in response to increased sputum volume or purulence and bronchodilator therapy increased to control symptoms.[47] Such interventions have been shown to reduce admission rates[82,83]; however, not all patients are suitable for these strategies. Patients with COPD are frequently elderly and may have cognitive difficulties limiting their ability to self manage, particularly when acutely unwell. Further research is required in this area, with a focus on identification and management of patients at high risk of hospital admission.[84]

Inhaled or Nebulized Bronchodilators

Bronchodilators relieve dyspnea and airflow obstruction during exacerbations[85] and short-acting inhaled β_2 agonists are usually the preferred bronchodilators for the initial treatment of COPD exacerbations.[86] The addition of anticholinergics has the potential for increased therapeutic benefit; however, empiric evidence to support this combination is lacking[85] and the drugs are generally reserved for exacerbations that exhibit a suboptimal response to inhaled β_2 agonists alone.[86] Nebulizers and hand-held inhalers can be used to administer inhaled bronchodilators during exacerbations of COPD and the choice of delivery method should consider the ability of the patient to use the device and the dose of drug required.[47]

Antibiotics

There is considerable evidence to support the role of bacteria in COPD exacerbation etiology and most guidelines highlight that antibiotics are beneficial in selected patients.[86] Purulent sputum is a reasonable surrogate of bacterial infection[27] and routine antibiotic use is normally advised only in the context of exacerbations associated with an increase in sputum purulence.[86] Much of the evidence for these recommendations stems from the seminal study by Anthonisen and colleagues[26] that provided strong evidence that antibiotics had a significant effect on peak expiratory flow rate (PEFR) and led to earlier resolution of symptoms. Type 1 exacerbations (those associated with increased sputum volume, sputum purulence, and dyspnea) benefited the most with resolution of symptoms in 63% of the antibiotic-treated exacerbations and 43% of the placebo group. However, patients with type 3 exacerbations (who met just one of the three cardinal symptoms) did not show significant benefit.

Studies have also assessed the benefits of stratifying antibiotic use according to exacerbation severity. However, the concept of exacerbation severity is difficult, reflecting the severity of the initiating insult, and that of the underlying COPD. In COPD exacerbations requiring mechanical ventilation, oral ofloxacin reduced in-hospital mortality, duration of hospital stay, length of mechanical ventilation, and the need for additional courses of antibiotics.[87] Therefore, in addition to exacerbations associated with increased sputum purulence, antibiotics are recommended in severe exacerbations requiring mechanical ventilation.[86]

The choice of antibiotics remains uncertain, predominantly because of methodologic limitations hampering comparison of studies examining different antibiotics. At present, most guidelines suggest initial empiric treatment should be in the form of an aminopenicillin, a macrolide, or a tetracycline, taking into account guidance from local microbiologists and in the light of local resistance patterns.[47] In hospitalized patients, sputum should be sent for culture at exacerbation if purulent, and the appropriateness of therapy checked against sensitivities when available. In those patients at high risk of _P aeruginosa_, fluoroquinolones should be considered.

Antiviral Agents

Viral infections (in particular rhinovirus) play a key role in exacerbation etiology and a variety of potential therapeutic agents have been trialed for the treatment of rhinoviral infections. Compounds have attempted to target cell susceptibility, viral attachment and receptor blockade, viral uncoating, viral RNA replication, and viral protein synthesis. Unfortunately, although the neuraminidase inhibitors amantadine and zanamivir are effective against influenza, antirhinoviral compounds have failed to demonstrate a clinically significant benefit in trials and are often complicated by adverse events and lack of tolerability.[88,89]

Systemic Corticosteroids

Multiple studies have found significant short-term benefits of corticosteroids in the treatment of COPD exacerbations. Corticosteroids lead to improvements in FEV_1 in the first 3 to 5 days of treatment[90–92] and Pao_2 in the first 72 hours compared with placebo.[92,93] Corticosteroids have also been shown to reduce hospitalization length[90,91] and the likelihood of treatment failure.[94] However, treatment of exacerbations with corticosteroids has not been shown to improve mortality.[94]

Considerable debate exists regarding the optimal dose and duration of treatment for acute exacerbations, often because of the heterogeneity of treatment regimens in different clinical trials.[95] There is no clear benefit of intravenous therapy over oral preparations and most guidelines recommend a dose of 30 to 40 mg oral prednisone per day for duration of 7 to 14 days.[47,86] There is no advantage in prolonged courses of therapy[91] and shorter courses of therapy reduce the risk of adverse effects. Tapering of this regimen is not required for most patients.[96] The most common reported adverse effect of corticosteroid therapy is hyperglycemia, particularly in patients with preexisting diabetes mellitus,[91] although osteoporosis prophylaxis should also be considered in patients requiring frequent courses of treatment.

The addition of antibiotics to oral steroids as part of exacerbation treatment may have further benefits to regimens composed of oral corticosteroids alone. Epidemiologic research using data from historical cohorts found that adding antibiotics to oral corticosteroids as part of index exacerbation treatment was associated with an increased time to the next exacerbation,[97] a reduced risk of future exacerbations, and reduced risk of all-cause mortality.[98]

Methylxanthines (Theophylline)

Intravenous theophyllines seem to increase respiratory drive, act as bronchodilators, and produce small improvements in acid–base balance during COPD exacerbations.[99] However, they do not improve lung function, dyspnea, or length of hospital stay when given in addition to nebulized bronchodilators and corticosteroids.[99] Given the toxicity associated with these medications, intravenous theophyllines are reserved for patients inadequately responding to standard therapy consisting of nebulized bronchodilators, oral corticosteroids, and antibiotics where indicated.

Oxygen

Oxygen is a treatment for hypoxemia, not breathlessness. However, when patients are hospitalized for exacerbations oxygen is not uncommonly administered during ambulance transportation, at assessment, and on admission. Oxygen must be prescribed with caution in this context because the respiratory drive of some patients with COPD may depend on their degree of hypoxia rather than the usual dependence on hypercapnia. Although rarely seen, overzealous and unmonitored oxygen therapy may result in suppression of a patient's respiratory drive, CO_2 narcosis, and respiratory arrest. Therefore, on arrival at the emergency room, arterial blood gases should be measured and the inspired oxygen concentration adjusted accordingly. Patients who have had a prior episode of hypercapnic respiratory failure should be issued with an oxygen alert card and a 24% or 28% Venturi mask for use during transportation.[47] For most patients with known COPD a target saturation range of 88% to 92% is recommended pending the availability of blood gas results.[100]

NIV

NIV, usually administered as pressure-cycled bi-level positive airway pressure is the treatment of choice for hypercapnic respiratory failure at acute exacerbation of COPD that persists despite optimal medical therapy including controlled oxygen therapy. NIV has been shown to improve gas exchange and acid–base disturbances. Consequently, NIV can reduce the length of hospital stay, mortality, and the need for intubation compared with usual medical care.[101] NIV should be delivered in a dedicated setting by trained, experienced staff. Before patients commence treatment, a clear management plan must be established to determine a course of action in the event of deterioration and to define the ceiling of care.[47]

Invasive Ventilation

If patients do not respond adequately or tolerate NIV (eg, because of multiorgan failure or reduced levels of consciousness), they may require endotracheal intubation and invasive ventilation. Historically, there has been a reluctance to intubate patients with COPD because of concerns about weaning and long-term outcomes. However, patients receiving mechanical ventilation because of acute decompensation of COPD have a significantly lower mortality (estimated 22%) than patients receiving mechanical ventilation for acute respiratory failure from other etiologies.[102] Thus, patients with exacerbations of COPD should be considered eligible to receive treatment on intensive care units, including invasive ventilation when necessary. Factors to be considered before admission include premorbid functional status, body mass index, the prevalence and severity of comorbidities, stable-state oxygen requirements, and prior intensive care unit admissions, in addition to age and degree of airflow obstruction or lung function impairment.[47]

Palliative Care

Palliative care involves the active care of patients and their families by a multidisciplinary team when a patient's disease is no longer responsive to curative treatment. Palliative care focuses on symptom control and optimizing quality of life. Anxiety and depression is common in COPD and may become particularly problematic in patients with end-stage disease, and those hospitalized with exacerbations. These symptoms should be treated with conventional pharmacotherapy. Intractable dyspnea that is unresponsive to other medical therapies may be treated with opiates, benzodiazepines, and tricyclic antidepressants[47]; however, there is little evidence to support the use of oxygen to relieve dyspnea in nonhypoxemic patients.[103] Palliative care should also include consideration of admission to hospices.

SUMMARY

The mechanisms of COPD exacerbation are complex. Respiratory viruses (in particular rhinovirus) and bacteria play a major role in the causative etiology of COPD exacerbations. In some patients, noninfective environmental factors may also be important. Data recently published from a large observational study identified a phenotype of patients more susceptible to frequent exacerbations. Many current therapeutic strategies can reduce exacerbation frequency. Future studies may target the frequent exacerbator phenotype, or those patients colonized with potential bacterial pathogens, for such therapies as long-term antibiotics, thus preventing exacerbations by decreasing bacterial load or preventing new strain acquisition in the stable state. Respiratory viral infections are also an important therapeutic target for COPD. Further work is required to develop new anti-inflammatory agents for exacerbation prevention, and novel acute treatments to improve outcomes at exacerbation.

REFERENCES

1. Burden of lung disease report. 2nd edition. British Thoracic Society (BTS); 2006. Available at: http://www.brit-thoracic.org.uk/Portals/0/Library/BTSPublications/burdeon_of_lung_disease2007.pdf. Accessed September 14, 2011.
2. Hurst JR, Vestbo J, Anzueto A, et al. Susceptibility to exacerbation in chronic obstructive pulmonary disease. N Engl J Med 2010;363(12):1128–38.
3. Donaldson GC, Seemungal TA, Bhowmik A, et al. Relationship between exacerbation frequency and lung function decline in chronic obstructive pulmonary disease. Thorax 2002;57(10):847–52.
4. Kanner RE, Anthonisen NR, Connett JE. Lower respiratory illnesses promote FEV(1) decline in current smokers but not ex-smokers with mild chronic obstructive pulmonary disease: results from the Lung Health Study. Am J Respir Crit Care Med 2001;164(3):358–64.
5. Donaldson GC, Hurst JR, Smith CJ, et al. Increased risk of myocardial infarction and stroke following exacerbation of COPD. Chest 2010;137(5):1091–7.
6. Seemungal TA, Donaldson GC, Paul EA, et al. Effect of exacerbation on quality of life in patients with chronic obstructive pulmonary disease. Am J Respir Crit Care Med 1998;157(5 Pt 1):1418–22.

7. Soler-Cataluna JJ, Martinez-Garcia MA, Roman Sanchez P, et al. Severe acute exacerbations and mortality in patients with chronic obstructive pulmonary disease. Thorax 2005;60(11):925–31.

8. Garcia-Aymerich J, Farrero E, Felez MA, et al. Risk factors of readmission to hospital for a COPD exacerbation: a prospective study. Thorax 2003;58(2): 100–5.

9. Burge S, Wedzicha JA. COPD exacerbations: definitions and classifications. Eur Respir J Suppl 2003;41:46s–53s.

10. Seemungal T, Harper-Owen R, Bhowmik A, et al. Respiratory viruses, symptoms, and inflammatory markers in acute exacerbations and stable chronic obstructive pulmonary disease. Am J Respir Crit Care Med 2001;164(9): 1618–23.

11. Bhowmik A, Seemungal TA, Sapsford RJ, et al. Relation of sputum inflammatory markers to symptoms and lung function changes in COPD exacerbations. Thorax 2000;55(2):114–20.

12. Seemungal TA, Donaldson GC, Bhowmik A, et al. Time course and recovery of exacerbations in patients with chronic obstructive pulmonary disease. Am J Respir Crit Care Med 2000;161(5):1608–13.

13. Rohde G, Wiethege A, Borg I, et al. Respiratory viruses in exacerbations of chronic obstructive pulmonary disease requiring hospitalisation: a case-control study. Thorax 2003;58(1):37–42.

14. Mallia P, Message SD, Gielen V, et al. Experimental rhinovirus infection as a human model of chronic obstructive pulmonary disease exacerbation. Am J Respir Crit Care Med 2011;183(6):734–42.

15. Schneider D, Ganesan S, Comstock AT, et al. Increased cytokine response of rhinovirus-infected airway epithelial cells in chronic obstructive pulmonary disease. Am J Respir Crit Care Med 2010;182(3):332–40.

16. Di Stefano A, Maestrelli P, Roggeri A, et al. Upregulation of adhesion molecules in the bronchial mucosa of subjects with chronic obstructive bronchitis. Am J Respir Crit Care Med 1994;149(3 Pt 1):803–10.

17. Donaldson GC, Seemungal T, Jeffries DJ, et al. Effect of temperature on lung function and symptoms in chronic obstructive pulmonary disease. Eur Respir J 1999;13(4):844–9.

18. Lyon JL, Stoddard G, Ferguson D, et al. An every other year cyclic epidemic of infants hospitalized with respiratory syncytial virus. Pediatrics 1996;97(1):152–3.

19. Meerhoff TJ, Paget JW, Kimpen JL, et al. Variation of respiratory syncytial virus and the relation with meteorological factors in different winter seasons. Pediatr Infect Dis J 2009;28(10):860–6.

20. Wilkinson TM, Donaldson GC, Johnston SL, et al. Respiratory syncytial virus, airway inflammation, and FEV1 decline in patients with chronic obstructive pulmonary disease. Am J Respir Crit Care Med 2006;173(8):871–6.

21. Nichol KL, Baken L, Nelson A. Relation between influenza vaccination and outpatient visits, hospitalization, and mortality in elderly persons with chronic lung disease. Ann Intern Med 1999;130(5):397–403.

22. Sethi S. Infectious etiology of acute exacerbations of chronic bronchitis. Chest 2000;117(5 Suppl 2):380S–5S.

23. Sethi S, Murphy TF. Bacterial infection in chronic obstructive pulmonary disease in 2000: a state-of-the-art review. Clin Microbiol Rev 2001;14(2):336–63.

24. Murphy TF, Brauer AL, Sethi S, et al. *Haemophilus haemolyticus*: a human respiratory tract commensal to be distinguished from *Haemophilus influenzae*. J Infect Dis 2007;195(1):81–9.

25. Sethi S, Evans N, Grant BJ, et al. New strains of bacteria and exacerbations of chronic obstructive pulmonary disease. N Engl J Med 2002;347(7):465–71.
26. Anthonisen NR, Manfreda J, Warren CP, et al. Antibiotic therapy in exacerbations of chronic obstructive pulmonary disease. Ann Intern Med 1987;106(2): 196–204.
27. Stockley RA, O'Brien C, Pye A, et al. Relationship of sputum color to nature and outpatient management of acute exacerbations of COPD. Chest 2000; 117(6):1638–45.
28. Miravitlles M, Marin A, Monso E, et al. Colour of sputum is a marker for bacterial colonisation in chronic obstructive pulmonary disease. Respir Res 2010; 11:58.
29. Monso E, Ruiz J, Rosell A, et al. Bacterial infection in chronic obstructive pulmonary disease. A study of stable and exacerbated outpatients using the protected specimen brush. Am J Respir Crit Care Med 1995;152(4 Pt 1):1316–20.
30. Patel IS, Seemungal TA, Wilks M, et al. Relationship between bacterial colonisation and the frequency, character, and severity of COPD exacerbations. Thorax 2002;57(9):759–64.
31. Hilty M, Burke C, Pedro H, et al. Disordered microbial communities in asthmatic airways. PLoS One 2010;5(1):e8578.
32. Erb-Downward JR, Thompson DL, Han MK, et al. Analysis of the lung microbiome in the "healthy" smoker and in COPD. PLoS One 2011;6(2):e16384.
33. Wilkinson TM, Hurst JR, Perera WR, et al. Effect of interactions between lower airway bacterial and rhinoviral infection in exacerbations of COPD. Chest 2006;129(2):317–24.
34. Rosell A, Monso E, Soler N, et al. Microbiologic determinants of exacerbation in chronic obstructive pulmonary disease. Arch Intern Med 2005;165(8):891–7.
35. Sethi S, Sethi R, Eschberger K, et al. Airway bacterial concentrations and exacerbations of chronic obstructive pulmonary disease. Am J Respir Crit Care Med 2007;176(4):356–61.
36. Abusriwil H, Stockley RA. Bacterial load and exacerbations of COPD. Am J Respir Crit Care Med 2008;177(9):1048–9 [author reply: 1049].
37. Sajjan US, Jia Y, Newcomb DC, et al. H. influenzae potentiates airway epithelial cell responses to rhinovirus by increasing ICAM-1 and TLR3 expression. FASEB J 2006;20(12):2121–3.
38. Papi A, Bellettato CM, Braccioni F, et al. Infections and airway inflammation in chronic obstructive pulmonary disease severe exacerbations. Am J Respir Crit Care Med 2006;173(10):1114–21.
39. Anderson HR, Spix C, Medina S, et al. Air pollution and daily admissions for chronic obstructive pulmonary disease in 6 European cities: results from the APHEA project. Eur Respir J 1997;10(5):1064–71.
40. Wordley J, Walters S, Ayres JG. Short term variations in hospital admissions and mortality and particulate air pollution. Occup Environ Med 1997;54(2):108–16.
41. Dominici F, Peng RD, Bell ML, et al. Fine particulate air pollution and hospital admission for cardiovascular and respiratory diseases. JAMA 2006;295(10): 1127–34.
42. Nordenhall C, Pourazar J, Blomberg A, et al. Airway inflammation following exposure to diesel exhaust: a study of time kinetics using induced sputum. Eur Respir J 2000;15(6):1046–51.
43. Rudell B, Blomberg A, Helleday R, et al. Bronchoalveolar inflammation after exposure to diesel exhaust: comparison between unfiltered and particle trap filtered exhaust. Occup Environ Med 1999;56(8):527–34.

44. Nichol KL, Nordin JD, Nelson DB, et al. Effectiveness of influenza vaccine in the community-dwelling elderly. N Engl J Med 2007;357(14):1373–81.
45. Nichol KL, Baken L, Wuorenma J, et al. The health and economic benefits associated with pneumococcal vaccination of elderly persons with chronic lung disease. Arch Intern Med 1999;159(20):2437–42.
46. Alfageme I, Vazquez R, Reyes N, et al. Clinical efficacy of anti-pneumococcal vaccination in patients with COPD. Thorax 2006;61(3):189–95.
47. National Clinical Guideline Centre. Chronic obstructive pulmonary disease: management of chronic obstructive pulmonary disease in adults in primary and secondary care. London: National Clinical Guideline Centre; 2010. Available at: http://guidance.nice.org.uk/CG101/Guidance/pdf/English. Accessed September 14, 2011.
48. Sprenkle MD, Niewoehner DE, MacDonald R, et al. Clinical efficacy of OM-85 BV in COPD and chronic bronchitis: a systematic review. COPD 2005;2(1):167–75.
49. Orcel B, Delclaux B, Baud M, et al. Oral immunization with bacterial extracts for protection against acute bronchitis in elderly institutionalized patients with chronic bronchitis. Eur Respir J 1994;7(3):446–52.
50. Collet JP, Shapiro P, Ernst P, et al. Effects of an immunostimulating agent on acute exacerbations and hospitalizations in patients with chronic obstructive pulmonary disease. The PARI-IS Study Steering Committee and Research Group. Prevention of Acute Respiratory Infection by an Immunostimulant. Am J Respir Crit Care Med 1997;156(6):1719–24.
51. Soler M, Mutterlein R, Cozma G. Double-blind study of OM-85 in patients with chronic bronchitis or mild chronic obstructive pulmonary disease. Respiration 2007;74(1):26–32.
52. Cazzola M, Rogliani P, Curradi G. Bacterial extracts for the prevention of acute exacerbations in chronic obstructive pulmonary disease: a point of view. Respir Med 2008;102(3):321–7.
53. Burge PS, Calverley PM, Jones PW, et al. Randomised, double blind, placebo controlled study of fluticasone propionate in patients with moderate to severe chronic obstructive pulmonary disease: the ISOLDE trial. BMJ 2000; 320(7245):1297–303.
54. Calverley PM, Anderson JA, Celli B, et al. Salmeterol and fluticasone propionate and survival in chronic obstructive pulmonary disease. N Engl J Med 2007; 356(8):775–89.
55. Tashkin DP, Celli B, Senn S, et al. A 4-year trial of tiotropium in chronic obstructive pulmonary disease. N Engl J Med 2008;359(15):1543–54.
56. Aaron SD, Vandemheen KL, Fergusson D, et al. Tiotropium in combination with placebo, salmeterol, or fluticasone-salmeterol for treatment of chronic obstructive pulmonary disease: a randomized trial. Ann Intern Med 2007;146(8): 545–55.
57. Puhan MA, Bachmann LM, Kleijnen J, et al. Inhaled drugs to reduce exacerbations in patients with chronic obstructive pulmonary disease: a network meta-analysis. BMC Med 2009;7:2.
58. Rossi A, Kristufek P, Levine BE, et al. Comparison of the efficacy, tolerability, and safety of formoterol dry powder and oral, slow-release theophylline in the treatment of COPD. Chest 2002;121(4):1058–69.
59. Zhou Y, Wang X, Zeng X, et al. Positive benefits of theophylline in a randomized, double-blind, parallel-group, placebo-controlled study of low-dose, slow-release theophylline in the treatment of COPD for 1 year. Respirology 2006; 11(5):603–10.

60. Calverley PM, Rabe KF, Goehring UM, et al. Roflumilast in symptomatic chronic obstructive pulmonary disease: two randomised clinical trials. Lancet 2009; 374(9691):685–94.
61. Seemungal TA, Wilkinson TM, Hurst JR, et al. Long-term erythromycin therapy is associated with decreased chronic obstructive pulmonary disease exacerbations. Am J Respir Crit Care Med 2008;178(11):1139–47.
62. Albert RK, Connett J, Bailey WC, et al. Azithromycin for prevention of exacerbations of COPD. N Engl J Med 2011;365(8):689–98.
63. Sethi S, Jones PW, Theron MS, et al. Pulsed moxifloxacin for the prevention of exacerbations of chronic obstructive pulmonary disease: a randomized controlled trial. Respir Res 2010;11:10.
64. Zheng JP, Kang J, Huang SG, et al. Effect of carbocisteine on acute exacerbation of chronic obstructive pulmonary disease (PEACE Study): a randomised placebo-controlled study. Lancet 2008;371(9629):2013–8.
65. Barnes PJ. Corticosteroid resistance in airway disease. Proc Am Thorac Soc 2004;1(3):264–8.
66. Ito K, Ito M, Elliott WM, et al. Decreased histone deacetylase activity in chronic obstructive pulmonary disease. N Engl J Med 2005;352(19):1967–76.
67. Cosio BG, Tsaprouni L, Ito K, et al. Theophylline restores histone deacetylase activity and steroid responses in COPD macrophages. J Exp Med 2004; 200(5):689–95.
68. Ito K, Lim S, Caramori G, et al. A molecular mechanism of action of theophylline: induction of histone deacetylase activity to decrease inflammatory gene expression. Proc Natl Acad Sci U S A 2002;99(13):8921–6.
69. Marwick JA, Caramori G, Casolari P, et al. A role for phosphoinositol 3-kinase delta in the impairment of glucocorticoid responsiveness in patients with chronic obstructive pulmonary disease. J Allergy Clin Immunol 2010;125(5):1146–53.
70. Marwick JA, Caramori G, Stevenson CS, et al. Inhibition of PI3Kdelta restores glucocorticoid function in smoking-induced airway inflammation in mice. Am J Respir Crit Care Med 2009;179(7):542–8.
71. Renda T, Baraldo S, Pelaia G, et al. Increased activation of p38 MAPK in COPD. Eur Respir J 2008;31(1):62–9.
72. Armstrong J, Harbron C, Lea S, et al. Synergistic effects of p38 mitogen-activated protein kinase inhibition with a corticosteroid in alveolar macrophages from patients with chronic obstructive pulmonary disease. J Pharmacol Exp Ther 2011;338(3):732–40.
73. Fishman A, Martinez F, Naunheim K, et al. A randomized trial comparing lung-volume-reduction surgery with medical therapy for severe emphysema. N Engl J Med 2003;348(21):2059–73.
74. Washko GR, Fan VS, Ramsey SD, et al. The effect of lung volume reduction surgery on chronic obstructive pulmonary disease exacerbations. Am J Respir Crit Care Med 2008;177(2):164–9.
75. Continuous or nocturnal oxygen therapy in hypoxemic chronic obstructive lung disease: a clinical trial. Nocturnal Oxygen Therapy Trial Group. Ann Intern Med 1980;93(3):391–8.
76. Long term domiciliary oxygen therapy in chronic hypoxic cor pulmonale complicating chronic bronchitis and emphysema. Report of the Medical Research Council Working Party. Lancet 1981;1(8222):681–6.
77. Garcia-Aymerich J, Monso E, Marrades RM, et al. Risk factors for hospitalization for a chronic obstructive pulmonary disease exacerbation. EFRAM study. Am J Respir Crit Care Med 2001;164(6):1002–7.

78. McEvoy RD, Pierce RJ, Hillman D, et al. Nocturnal non-invasive nasal ventilation in stable hypercapnic COPD: a randomised controlled trial. Thorax 2009;64(7): 561–6.
79. Casaburi R, ZuWallack R. Pulmonary rehabilitation for management of chronic obstructive pulmonary disease. N Engl J Med 2009;360(13):1329–35.
80. Hurst JR, Wedzicha JA. Management and prevention of chronic obstructive pulmonary disease exacerbations: a state of the art review. BMC Med 2009;7: 40.
81. Wilkinson TM, Donaldson GC, Hurst JR, et al. Early therapy improves outcomes of exacerbations of chronic obstructive pulmonary disease. Am J Respir Crit Care Med 2004;169(12):1298–303.
82. Bourbeau J, Julien M, Maltais F, et al. Reduction of hospital utilization in patients with chronic obstructive pulmonary disease: a disease-specific self-management intervention. Arch Intern Med 2003;163(5):585–91.
83. Casas A, Troosters T, Garcia-Aymerich J, et al. Integrated care prevents hospitalisations for exacerbations in COPD patients. Eur Respir J 2006;28(1):123–30.
84. Wedzicha JA, Seemungal TA. COPD exacerbations: defining their cause and prevention. Lancet 2007;370(9589):786–96.
85. McCrory DC, Brown CD. Anti-cholinergic bronchodilators versus beta2-sympathomimetic agents for acute exacerbations of chronic obstructive pulmonary disease. Cochrane Database Syst Rev 2002;4:CD003900.
86. Global Strategy for the Diagnosis, Management and Prevention of COPD. Global Initiative for Chronic Obstructive Lung Disease (GOLD); 2009. Available at: http://www.goldcopd.org. Accessed September 14, 2011.
87. Nouira S, Marghli S, Belghith M, et al. Once daily oral ofloxacin in chronic obstructive pulmonary disease exacerbation requiring mechanical ventilation: a randomised placebo-controlled trial. Lancet 2001;358(9298):2020–5.
88. Martinez FJ. Pathogen-directed therapy in acute exacerbations of chronic obstructive pulmonary disease. Proc Am Thorac Soc 2007;4(8):647–58.
89. Anzueto A, Niederman MS. Diagnosis and treatment of rhinovirus respiratory infections. Chest 2003;123(5):1664–72.
90. Davies L, Angus RM, Calverley PM. Oral corticosteroids in patients admitted to hospital with exacerbations of chronic obstructive pulmonary disease: a prospective randomised controlled trial. Lancet 1999;354(9177):456–60.
91. Niewoehner DE, Erbland ML, Deupree RH, et al. Effect of systemic glucocorticoids on exacerbations of chronic obstructive pulmonary disease. Department of Veterans Affairs Cooperative Study Group. N Engl J Med 1999;340(25): 1941–7.
92. Thompson WH, Nielson CP, Carvalho P, et al. Controlled trial of oral prednisone in outpatients with acute COPD exacerbation. Am J Respir Crit Care Med 1996; 154(2 Pt 1):407–12.
93. Maltais F, Ostinelli J, Bourbeau J, et al. Comparison of nebulized budesonide and oral prednisolone with placebo in the treatment of acute exacerbations of chronic obstructive pulmonary disease: a randomized controlled trial. Am J Respir Crit Care Med 2002;165(5):698–703.
94. Wood-Baker RR, Gibson PG, Hannay M, et al. Systemic corticosteroids for acute exacerbations of chronic obstructive pulmonary disease. Cochrane Database Syst Rev 2005;1:CD001288.
95. McCrory DC, Brown C, Gray RN, et al. Management of acute exacerbations of chronic obstructive pulmonary disease. Evid Rep Technol Assess (Summ) 2000;(19):1–4.

96. Joint Formulary Committee. British National Formulary. 61st edition. London: British Medical Association and Royal Pharmaceutical Society; 2011.
97. Roede BM, Bresser P, Bindels PJ, et al. Antibiotic treatment is associated with reduced risk of a subsequent exacerbation in obstructive lung disease: an historical population based cohort study. Thorax 2008;63(11):968–73.
98. Roede BM, Bresser P, Prins JM, et al. Reduced risk of next exacerbation and mortality associated with antibiotic use in COPD. Eur Respir J 2009;33(2):282–8.
99. Duffy N, Walker P, Diamantea F, et al. Intravenous aminophylline in patients admitted to hospital with non-acidotic exacerbations of chronic obstructive pulmonary disease: a prospective randomised controlled trial. Thorax 2005; 60(9):713–7.
100. O'Driscoll BR, Howard LS, Davison AG. BTS guideline for emergency oxygen use in adult patients. Thorax 2008;63(Suppl 6):vi1–68.
101. Ram FS, Lightowler JV, Wedzicha JA. Non-invasive positive pressure ventilation for treatment of respiratory failure due to exacerbations of chronic obstructive pulmonary disease. Cochrane Database Syst Rev 2003;1:CD004104.
102. Esteban A, Anzueto A, Frutos F, et al. Characteristics and outcomes in adult patients receiving mechanical ventilation: a 28-day international study. JAMA 2002;287(3):345–55.
103. Clemens KE, Quednau I, Klaschik E. Use of oxygen and opioids in the palliation of dyspnoea in hypoxic and non-hypoxic palliative care patients: a prospective study. Support Care Cancer 2009;17(4):367–77.

Index

Note: Page numbers of article titles are in **boldface** type.

Immunol Allergy Clin N Am 33 (2013) 117–123
http://dx.doi.org/10.1016/S0889-8561(12)00158-0   **immunology.theclinics.com**
0889-8561/13/$ – see front matter © 2013 Elsevier Inc. All rights reserved.

Moving?

Make sure your subscription moves with you!

To notify us of your new address, find your **Clinics Account Number** (located on your mailing label above your name), and contact customer service at:

Email: journalscustomerservice-usa@elsevier.com

800-654-2452 (subscribers in the U.S. & Canada)
314-447-8871 (subscribers outside of the U.S. & Canada)

Fax number: 314-447-8029

**Elsevier Health Sciences Division
Subscription Customer Service
3251 Riverport Lane
Maryland Heights, MO 63043**

*To ensure uninterrupted delivery of your subscription, please notify us at least 4 weeks in advance of move.

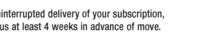

Printed and bound by CPI Group (UK) Ltd, Croydon, CR0 4YY

03/10/2024

01040443-0015